How to Validate a Pharmaceutical Process

How to Validate a Pharmaceutical Process

Steven A. Ostrove, PhD
President, Ostrove Associates, Inc.,
Elizabeth, NJ, United States

AMSTERDAM • BOSTON • HEIDELBERG • LONDON
NEW YORK • OXFORD • PARIS • SAN DIEGO
SAN FRANCISCO • SINGAPORE • SYDNEY • TOKYO

Academic Press is an imprint of Elsevier

Academic Press is an imprint of Elsevier
125 London Wall, London EC2Y 5AS, UK
525 B Street, Suite 1800, San Diego, CA 92101-4495, USA
50 Hampshire Street, 5th Floor, Cambridge, MA 02139, USA
The Boulevard, Langford Lane, Kidlington, Oxford OX5 1GB, UK

ISBN: 978-0-12-804148-2

Library of Congress Cataloging-in-Publication Data
A catalog record for this book is available from the Library of Congress

British Library Cataloguing-in-Publication Data
A catalogue record for this book is available from the British Library

For Information on all Academic Press publications
visit our website at http://www.elsevier.com/

Working together
to grow libraries in
developing countries

www.elsevier.com • www.bookaid.org

Publisher: Mica Haley
Acquisition Editor: Kristine Jones
Editorial Project Manager: Tracy I. Tufaga
Production Project Manager: Anusha Sambamoorthy
Designer: Mark Rogers

Typeset by MPS Limited, Chennai, India

DEDICATION

This book is dedicated to my wife, Karen. Without her love and support over my years in the industry, and on the road, this book would never have been possible.

CONTENTS

Author Biography.. xi
Preface.. xiii
Acknowledgment xv
About the *Expertise in the Pharmaceutical Process*
Technology Series xvii

SECTION I: INTRODUCTION TO PROCESS VALIDATION

Chapter 1 Introduction to Process Validation (PV)...............................3
Defining Process Validation (PV) 3
Legacy Products 7
Stages of PV 9
Notes 13

Chapter 2 A Brief Review of the Regulations.....................................15
Notes 30

Chapter 3 The Validation Life Cycle and Change Control.................33
Life Cycle Approach...33
The Role of Change Control 35
Types of Changes 37
The Change Control Process 40
Notes 41

SECTION II: STAGE I—PROCESS DEVELOPMENT

Chapter 4 Getting Started 45
Before It All Starts 45
Getting Started (After the Equipment Specifications)..........................47
The Validation Master Plan 48
Standard Operating Procedures (SOPs) Preparation...........................52
Quality Programs...53
Training...53

Basic Risk Approach 54
Putting it Together...55
Notes 58

Chapter 5 Basic Equipment and Utility Qualification 59
Introduction...59
Determining the Level of Qualification 60
Factory Acceptance Test and Site Acceptance Test..................60
Commissioning 62
Qualification Protocols—Installation Qualification (IQ)
and Operational Qualification (OQ)...64
Laboratory Equipment Qualification (EQ)................................67
Qualification Protocol Execution..68
Notes 70

Chapter 6 Computers and Automated Systems 71
Introduction...71
General Considerations 73
Specific Systems..79
Part 11 84
Notes 86

SECTION III: STAGE II—PROCESS DEVELOPMENT

Chapter 7 Process Development..89
Preliminaries 89
Development..90
Risk Assessment 93
Process Parameters 97
Setting Process Limits...99
Next Steps..101
Notes 102

Chapter 8 The Process Validation Protocol—PPQ 103
Introduction...103
Setting Protocol Test Ranges..104
Preparing the Protocol...106
Executing the Protocol...109
Notes 112

Chapter 9 Dealing With Deviations **113**
The Investigation 117
Notes 117

SECTION IV: STAGE III—CONTINUED PROCESS
            VERIFICATION

Chapter 10 Stage III—Collection and Evaluating Production Data ... 121
General Approach 121
Legacy Products 123
Stage III—Continued Process Verification (CPV) 125
Statistical Process Control and Control Charts 126
Notes 129

SECTION V: OTHER RELATED ACTIVITIES

Chapter 11 Cleaning and Facility Qualification **133**
Facility Design.. 133
Introduction to Cleaning 136
General Cleaning Considerations 136
Facility Design and Cleaning... 137
Equipment Cleaning 138
Other Cleaning Considerations.. 139
Notes 140

Terms and Definitions **141**
Appendix A: 21 CFR 211 ....**153**
Appendix B: Example—Short Change Control Form **191**
Appendix C: Additional ICH and FDA Guidelines **193**
Index..**195**

Steven A. Ostrove, PhD

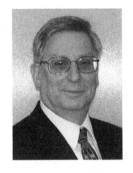

Steven Ostrove, President of Ostrove Associates, Inc. (OAI) provides validation and compliance consulting services to the Bio/Pharm industry. In 1999, Dr. Ostrove opened OAI in order to provide more personalized services to industry. He brings over 35 years of industry experience to OAI. OAI services include: start-up commissioning and validation; remediation for FDA warning letters and consent decrees. OAI specializes in process validation, cleaning validation, and computer system qualifications.

Dr. Ostrove has a PhD from Rutgers University in Biochemistry, a Masters in Biology from Adelphi University, and a Bachelors in Biology/Chemistry from SUNY Albany. He started his career as a research biochemist at Merck; and, after three years of postdoctoral work (Mt. Sinai School of Medicine and Columbia University— Harkness Eye Institute) in biochemistry, he moved to a technical service position at Pharmacia Biotech where he became the Manager of Computer Systems. With this experience, he then joined a major engineering design company and started the corporate validation— regulatory department. Moves to other major Architectural and Engineering firms resulted in his leading and reorganizing the Validation—Regulatory Affairs department for two additional firms.

Dr. Ostrove has over 25 publications, including six book chapters, on a wide variety of topics, ranging from Affinity Chromatography to Process Validation Scale-Up. He has been a course leader and organizer of training programs for ISPE and an invited lecturer by Pharma, PDA, and others. He has served on the exam preparation committee for ISPE's CPIP certification program and is currently a course director for three courses for the Center for Progressive

Innovative Education (CGMPs, QC Lab GMPs, and Process Validation). He has also served as an Adjunct Professor of Pharmaceutical Engineering at New Jersey Institute of Technology (Validation and Regulatory Affairs) and as an Adjunct Professor of Biology at Kean University (Biology). He recently completed service on an FDA advisory panel as the industry representative and received a service award for his tenure and contribution to the committee.

There have been many books written about utility and equipment qualification as well as process validation. All of these books and articles describe the technical inner workings of the various pieces of process equipment or systems. These are helpful, but they do not tell you how to move forward from there.

In performing a complete process validation program it is important to not only know what to do or what not to do but also to know why you are doing it. Thus, the goal of this book is to lead you through the workings of a successful process validation program. It includes those aspects of the surrounding operations that are necessary to complete the validation and attain full compliance to the Food and Drug Administration (FDA) Current Good Manufacturing Practices (CGMP) as found in the Code of Federal Regulations (CFR) Title 21 Parts 210 and 211.

This book is about preparing for and performing an acceptable process validation (PV) program for either new or legacy products. Notice, I again mention that it is a "program." This is because process validation is more than just verifying that the process is reproducible and reliable. There are many components, steps, and systems that are involved. For example, the process equipment must be qualified, the automation system(s) must be validated and meet Part 11 requirements, and laboratory methods need to be validated, etc. Another aspect that is critical to all compliance studies is maintaining data integrity. As you can see, performing a compliant PV takes a lot of work and time. It is important to show why things are done so that the operations are maintained within their control settings as well as their actual functioning.

By understanding the reasons for each step, understanding why things need to be recorded and how they need to be recorded, understanding the variables of the process and how they can be controlled (if at all), and the reasons why they are variable will allow you to comply with current FDA expectations and your own satisfaction that your product is safe and reproducible (ie, in control at all stages and if something was to go wrong you will be able to quickly mend the problem and get back into full compliance). This is not only good business but it is good manufacturing practice (GMP).

Steven A. Ostrove
Ostrove Associates, Inc.

ACKNOWLEDGMENT

I would like to thank Dr. Ken Blashka for his thoughtful discussions and his very helpful review of this manuscript. His comments and suggestions were extremely helpful in preparing the book.

Numerous books and articles have been published on the subject of pharmaceutical process technology. While most of them cover the subject matter in depth and include detailed descriptions of the processes and associated theories and practices of operations, there seems to be a significant lack of practical guides and "how to" publications.

The *Expertise in the Pharmaceutical Process Technology* series is designed to fill this void. It comprises volumes on specific subjects with case studies and practical advice on how to overcome challenges that the practitioners in various fields of pharmaceutical technology are facing.

FORMAT

- The series volumes will be published under the Elsevier Academic Press imprint in both paperback and electronic versions. Electronic versions will be full color, while print books will be published in black and white.

SUBJECT MATTER

- The series will be a collection of hands-on practical guides for practitioners with numerous case studies and step-by-step instructions for proper procedures and problem solving. Each topic will start with a brief overview of the subject matter and include an exposé, as well as practical solutions of the most common problems along with a lot of common sense (proven scientific rather than empirical practices).
- The series will try to avoid theoretical aspects of the subject matter and limit scientific/mathematical exposé (eg, modeling, finite elements computations, academic studies, review of publications, theoretical aspects of process physics or chemistry) unless absolutely vital for understanding or justification of practical approach as advocated by the volume author. At best, it will combine both the practical ("how to") and scientific ("why") approach, based on

practically proven solid theory–model–measurements. The main focus will be to ensure that a practitioner can use the recommended step-by-step approach to improve the results of his or her daily activities.

TARGET AUDIENCE

- The primary audience includes pharmaceutical personnel, from R&D and production technicians to team leaders and department heads. Some topics will also be of interest to people working in nutraceutical and generic manufacturing companies. The series will also be useful for those in academia and regulatory agencies. Each book in the series will target a specific audience.
- The Expertise in the *Pharmaceutical Process Technology* series presents concise, affordable, practical volumes that are valuable to patrons of pharmaceutical libraries as well as practitioners.

Welcome to the brave new world of practical guides to pharmaceutical technology!

Michael Levin, PhD
Milev, LLC Pharmaceutical Technology Consulting

Introduction to Process Validation

CHAPTER *1*

Introduction to Process Validation (PV)

DEFINING PROCESS VALIDATION (PV)

In order to correctly perform and complete a process validation (PV) one needs to be able to first define the process. Once an acceptable definition is available, then one needs to be able to act on it. PV is not mentioned in the current GMP regulations (21 CFR Part 211[1]). However, it is well defined in the 1987[2] and 2011[3] PV guidelines published by the Food and Drug Administration (FDA). As seen in the two definitions below, the FDA is concerned with documentation and consistency. In fact, in 1996 the FDA published in the Federal Register a proposed change to 21 CFR 211. They added a section on PV (Subpart L).[4] These changes were never implemented and the proposed changes (including Subparts L & M) were withdrawn. However, the definitions presented there were the same as those found in the 1987 guideline.

According to the FDA in their original guideline on PV[5] in 1987 (emphasis added by the author) the definition is:

> *Documented Evidence that provides a HIGH DEGREE OF ASSURANCE that a process will consistently operate or produce a product meeting its predetermined specifications and quality attributes.*

According to the current (2011) PV guideline[6] the definition is:

> *... the collection and evaluation of data, from the process design stage throughout production, which establishes scientific evidence that a process is capable of consistently delivering quality products.*

Note the similarity in the definitions. In the 1987 version the FDA refers to "documented evidence," while in the 2011 edition it refers to "the collection and evaluation of data." Both definitions refer to the same thing. Process data, or information obtained during the production process need to be collected, evaluated, and recorded. In addition, both call for consistency in operation and product quality attributes. The difference between the two definitions is that the

How to Validate a Pharmaceutical Process. DOI: http://dx.doi.org/10.1016/B978-0-12-804148-2.00001-9

1987 version refers to predetermined specifications, while the 2011 version refers to the process design stage throughout production. Again, the same things are stated but in different words. The predetermined specifications refer to determining the process quality attributes before the process is validated; in the 2011 version this is part of the process design stage (Stage I). The process design stage (Stage I) is where the predetermined attributes are established. This is further addressed in Chapter 7, "Process Development."

Several years passed between the first and current versions of the guideline. As already discussed, the first approach the FDA made to establish a recognized approach to PV was in 1987. Thus, shortly after the Current Good Manufacturing Practices (CGMPs) were introduced (1978) the FDA felt it necessary to define their requirements for a compliant PV. Note that in 1987 the FDA required a "high degree of assurance," not a guarantee, that the process will be consistent and meeting predetermined attributes. Today the FDA requires the evaluation of data on a scientific basis so as to assure that the product is consistent in maintaining its quality attributes (again not a guarantee). This is the same intent that they had back in 1987. The data should show a tight and consistent "fit" to the predetermined specifications over time. Thus, through the evaluation of the data over time you will gain a high degree of assurance that the product is consistently produced and meets its expected quality attributes.

Another way of looking at the definitions above is that this means that by following the scientific method for product development, quality will be built in to the process and not just tested at the end. This leads to the FDA's position paper on GMPs for the 21st century.[7] In this paper the FDA lays out the expectations for the risk-based approach to qualification and validation. In addition to the "risk" aspect, there is also a need for the process to demonstrate a good scientific approach. Together, these methods will allow the establishment of a defendable validation strategy. Several organizations (eg, ISPE, PDA, ASQ) have publications[8] dealing with the risk-based approach to validation.

Risk, as used by the FDA and the pharmaceutical industry, is taken to mean the risk to the patient. The industry needs to be aware of how each step of the production process impacts the final product and thus how it will impact the end user, the patient.

In simple terms, the greater the equipment impacts (or controls) the process, the more testing will be needed. Defining the risk involved in the process will be discussed in Chapters 4, "Getting Started" and 7, "Process Development."

Looking at the 2011 definition again, we see that we also need "scientific evidence" that the process and thus the product are consistent and effective as determined during development. Here, the FDA relies on using the scientific method for development and scale up. Testing is done for one variable at a time. Again, employment of a risk-based approach should be used in determining the tests to be conducted.

The PV is usually viewed as the "last" major step in reaching full compliance as found in the FDA guideline on PV (2011).[9] Note that "compliance" is referred to here, not "validation." The current approach is to compliance, which is meeting all parts of the CGMPs (21 CFR 211).[10] Figs. 1.1 and 1.2 outline the "old" and "new" approach to meeting the current FDA requirements.

It must be understood that maintaining compliance is a never-ending process. PV is not one step, thus it really isn't the "last step" in the compliance program (refer to Fig. 1.2) meeting the compliant state is a circle (thus a life cycle approach is needed). There are many pieces that need to come together before it can be considered complete. While this book is about developing a successful PV, other areas that support or otherwise contribute to the PV need to be considered.

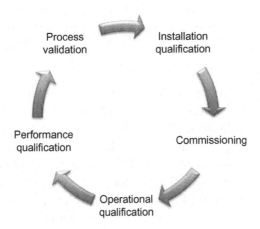

*Figure 1.1 Original approach = **VALIDATION**.*

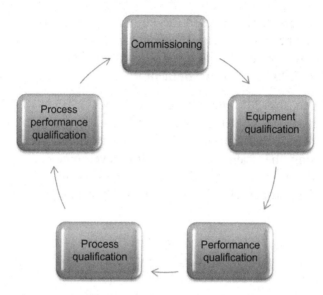

*Figure 1.2 Current approach = **COMPLIANCE**.*

For example, cleaning validation or the qualification of the facility are critical components of the PV. A manufacturer cannot just run their process without first assuring that all of the equipment, utilities, facility, and supporting processes are fully qualified or validated.[11] These are discussed in the later chapters.

The facility must be capable of producing the product (ie, its location, size, design). The equipment and utilities supporting the process need to be qualified and shown to meet the criteria needed to consistently produce the product (system suitability) and the operators need training on the process and use of the equipment. And lastly, but certainly not least, all aspects of 21 CFR 211 (GMPs for Finished Pharmaceuticals) must be met.

The CGMPs are written so as to allow the manufacturer the ability to control their own process. As you will find in Chapter 2, "A Brief Review of the Regulations," the regulations in Title 21 PART 211 of the Code of Federal Regulations (CFR) or in the Food, Drug, and Cosmetic Act (FD&C)[12] are not specific for PV. However, all of the rules apply even to non-pharmaceutical products (eg, biologics, devices, etc.). There are parts of the CFR that apply to other types of products yet Part 211 applies to all at least to some degree. Thus, if the manufacturing process is to produce a combination product Part 211 and the specific

Part for the combination product (eg, a stent containing a drug would follow 21 CFR 211 and 820) will be applicable.

There are four types of validation that can be performed. These are:

- Prospective—Preplanned tests with acceptance criteria that are measurable and prove that the production is reproducible.
- Concurrent[13]—In special situations the product will be released prior to demonstrating full reproducibility. It is still a preplanned test with acceptance criteria that are measurable. The FDA expects this type of validation approach to be rarely used. For example, it is not practical to produce a diagnostic radioactive tracer with a short half-life three or more times before the half-life loss would limit its use. Thus, it can be manufactured, tested, and sold prior to completing the requisite number of batches to complete a "full validation."
- Retrospective—Using existing products' data to support the validation effort.
- Revalidation—This is necessary only when a product is made in one facility then transferred to another or if there is a change in the process or process equipment that may alter its compliant state.

At this time the FDA expects that all validations are to be prospective, that is having preplanned acceptance criteria that must be met before the validation is considered complete and successful. The FDA expects all processes to be prospectively validated, however, now using only the new guideline.[14,15]

LEGACY PRODUCTS

For new products—those reaching the PV stage after Jan. 2011—following the current guideline should not be a problem. All stages need to be fully developed, written down, and documented that they have been performed as written. However, if a product was validated prior to the Jan. 2011 release of the current guideline (a legacy product) it may be necessary to review the information collected during what is now Stage I (process development) and "beef up" the development data. The question now becomes "What do I do with my existing processes?" For legacy products (those either in production prior to Jan. 2011 or having completed the PV stage prior to the date of promulgation) the work usually starts in Stage III.

The answer is, all manufacturing must now meet the requirements outlined in the new PV guideline. Thus, for a legacy product it is generally accepted to start with a Stage III review of the Critical Process Parameters (CPPs) and Critical Quality Attributes (CQAs) for the existing process. Each manufacturer has differing amounts of information regarding each of these stages for existing product manufacturing. Fig. 1.3 is a flowchart outlining the approach needed in the evaluation of a legacy product.

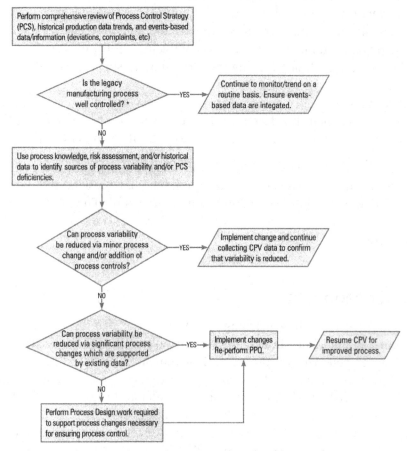

* Is an appropriate Process Control Strategy (demonstrating understanding of the impact of process parameters on CQAs) defined and does statistical of data show that variability is controlled?

Figure 1.3 CPV plan for legacy products. Source: PDA TR60 with permission.[14]

In order to bring current processes into line with the current guideline the following steps can be taken.

1. Follow all corporate change control and documentation procedures
2. Where and when possible collect the development data for each product
   a. Review the scientific literature related to the process
      i. Has anything changed?
      ii. Any improvements in the chemistry?
   b. Perform additional testing where the original work is felt to be weak of incomplete
3. Reevaluate the CPPs and CQAs
   a. Are they still critical?
   b. Are they all necessary?
   c. Are any other steps now found to be "critical?"
4. Any change made to the process should be fully developed and tested prior to implementation regardless of how minor it is considered. For example:
   a. Line speed adjustments even within "validated ranges"
   b. Cleaning conditions

STAGES OF PV

The new guideline presents three stages for the completion of the PV. These are:

Stage I—Process Development
- The utility, equipment, and facilities qualification
- Establishing critical parameters
  - CPPs
  - CQAs
- Development of Other Quality Systems or Programs
  - Computer Systems
  - Cleaning Verification
  - Change Control
  - Preventive Maintenance and Calibration

Stage II—Process Qualification
- Setting up the validation tests
- Documenting the process fulfills its preestablished criteria consistently (ie, sufficient batches run and tested)
- Handling (resolving) Deviations

Stage III—Continued Process Verification
- Control Charts for CPPs/CQAs
- Annual Product Reports (APRs)
- Statistical Evaluation of the data
  - C_p/C_{pk}
  - P_k/P_{pk}

Stage I (as further discussed in Chapter 7: Process Development) includes not just obtaining information about the potential drug product, but also developing the validation approach (ie, preparing the validation master plan, vendor selection, equipment specification, and more).

Stage II (as further discussed in Chapter 8: The Process Validation Protocol—PPQ) covers what was known as the PV in the 1987 guideline. Under the new guideline it is referred to as the Process Performance Qualification or PPQ. This is where the manufacturer runs the process as developed in Stage I (and scale up development) several times to prove that the process can be maintained in control over time. This stage is usually the best-documented stage when faced with qualifying existing products. The FDA understands that preexisting processes do not necessarily meet current requirements, in particular Stage I. However, Stage II is usually well documented since PV has been in effect at least since 1978 and defined in 1987. Current manufacturers even have some of Stage III as presented in the APRs. While the goal is to fully comply with the new guideline, companies are struggling to do so.

Stage III (as further discussed in Chapter 10: Stage III—Collection and Evaluating Production Data) provides ongoing proof that the product's production, and any continuous improvements that are made, remain in control and a consistent product is produced. This stage is not just a follow up to the PPQ; it is a full component of the PV. Thus, the three-batch paradigm is no longer viable. As specified in the guideline, "a sufficient number of batches" are needed to demonstrate control and consistency. The manufacturer needs to determine how many batches will be needed (statistical evaluation is important) to be assured that the production is in control and consistent.

Based on the new guideline, it should be apparent that other functions are to be included in the validation process. The FDA is concerned with process control (automation and computer systems)

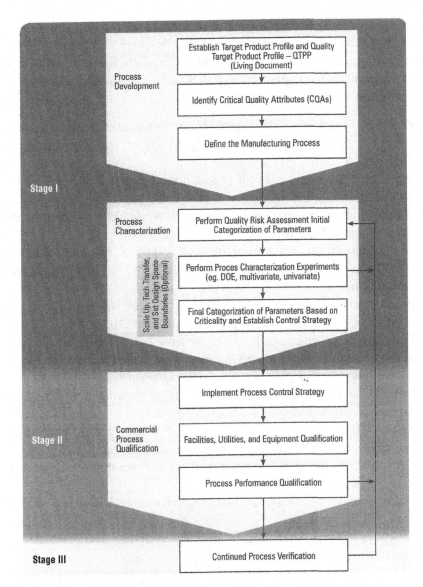

Figure 1.4 Summary of activities for CGMP compliance. Source: PDA TR60 with permission.[14]

(see Chapter 6: Computers and Automated Systems), data integrity (see Chapter 10: Stage III—Collection and Evaluating Production Data), cleaning and facilities (see Chapter 11: Cleaning and Facility Qualification).

Fig. 1.4 is a flowchart of the pathway that is needed to reach compliance. It outlines the main events to be included in a PV.

Note that each of the steps can be further broken down into smaller units. From this diagram, it can be understood that completing a PV is complicated, yet easy to perform. The main points that are stressed by the FDA and other regulatory agencies for a successful and complete PV program are:

- Provide a good scientific approach and rationale for all considerations (eg, specification development, equipment sizing, computer or automation control functions, etc.).
- Perform a risk analysis of all production steps and of all equipment and utilities.
- Assure that all process equipment are fully qualified and meet the requirements of the process.
- Assure that all process utilities are qualified or at least commissioned (based on a risk assessment and extent of product contact or interaction).
- Be assured that the facility is capable of safely manufacturing the product (ie, environmental conditions can be met).
- Understanding your product—know how each step in the process of the product is controlled and why the step needs to be controlled.
- Demonstrate reproducibility—be able to set reasonable and realistic ranges for production.
- Know what causes variation—determine the factors that cause increases or decreases in the product's attributes (not just CQAs).
- Demonstrate that each of the critical control points are successfully tested—measure each CQA.
- Qualify and/or validate related ancillary and necessary CGMP and quality programs (eg, calibration and preventative maintenance programs, cleaning, computer systems, and automation controls).

The emphasis in this book is on the 2011 PV guideline. However, other supporting information will be presented so as to provide a clearer picture of how to validate a pharmaceutical process. While not specifically covered, biologics and devices do follow a similar route to compliance. By understanding the process and all the aspects that control the chemistry and physical properties, a product will meet the current expectations of all regulatory agencies. All of this will be discussed in more detail throughout the book.

NOTES

1. Title 21 Code of Federal Regulations Parts 210 and 211, 2015.

2. Guideline on General Principles of Process Val, FDA, 1987.

3. Guidance for Industry Process Validation: General Principles and Practices, FDA, Jan. 2011.

4. Federal Resister, May 3, 1996 FDA, 21 CFR 210 and 211, Proposed Rule.

5. Guideline on General Principles of Process Val, FDA, 1987.

6. Guidance for Industry Process Validation: General Principles and Practices, FDA, Jan. 2011.

7. Pharmaceutical CGMPs for the 21st Century—A Risk-Based Approach Final Report; FDA, Sep. 2004.

8. www.PDA.org, www.ISPE.org, www.ASQ.org

9. Guidance for Industry Process Validation: General Principles and Practices, FDA, Jan. 2011.

10. Guidance for Industry Process Validation: General Principles and Practices, FDA, Jan. 2011.

11. NOTE: for this book we will refer to the paradigm that equipment is qualified and processes are validated.

12. Federal Food, Drug, and Cosmetic Act; Apr. 24, 2013.

13. Guidance for Industry Process Validation: General Principles and Practices, FDA, Jan. 2011, p. 16.

14. Technical Report No. 60; Process Validation: A Life Cycle Approach, Parenteral Drug Association, 2013.

15. Technical Report No. 60-2; Process Validation: A Life Cycle Approach—OSD/SSD Annex, Parenteral Drug Association, In Press.

CHAPTER 2

A Brief Review of the Regulations*

The US Food and Drug Administration (FDA) expects that pharmaceutical manufacturers follow the rules set forth to assure a quality product. With this, they expect that quality be built into the product, not tested into the product. This is the basis for the Quality by Design or QbD program.[1] The law that governs the pharmaceutical industry is the Food, Drug, and Cosmetic Act (FD&C). This was originally promulgated in 1906 and revised over time. From this set of laws the FDA is authorized to establish and publish rules that support the FD&C. This is in the Code of Federal Regulations (CFR) Title 21. Parts 210 and 211 are known as the Good Manufacturing Practices (GMPs) for Finished Pharmaceuticals. As will be seen, the GMPs are interpretive, allowing the manufacturer to implement them as necessary for their product(s). Meeting the GMP requirements is not only necessary but also makes good business sense. The reason for this is that in any business one needs to know that the equipment and materials purchased are the ones specified and that they will all perform as expected. If they do not, there can be great losses to the company.

In this chapter some of the key regulations that pertain to process validation will be reviewed. The selected regulations presented here are considered key to completing a successful process validation. Nonetheless, all of the other GMPs need to be reviewed and adhered to during the design and implementation of the process validation program (see Appendix A for the complete 21 CFR 211). In addition, some of the guidelines promulgated by the FDA are also reviewed. While not binding for the industry, these guidelines make good sense for meeting the expectations of the regulatory agencies.

Chapter 5 of the FD&C act deals with pharmaceuticals. Section 501(a)(2)(B) of the act defines adulterated products and is the basis for the FDA's authority.

In addition to the documents and regulations summarized here, the FDA provides many guideline documents that should be referred to before

---

*Bold text in this chapter is by the author for clarity only.

How to Validate a Pharmaceutical Process. DOI: http://dx.doi.org/10.1016/B978-0-12-804148-2.00002-0

a process validation is started (eg, The process Validation Guideline,[2] Q7,[3] Guide to Cleaning Validations,[4] and many more—refer to the list in Appendix C). Along with the FDA guidelines the International Conference on Harmonization (ICH)[5] also has a series of guidelines (also in Appendix C) to help understand and comply with all of the requirements of pharmaceutical manufacturing. These guidelines when fully approved by all parties (United States, EU, and Japan) become FDA guidance documents.

In particular, there are three ICH guidelines that deserve special attention for preparing and for executing a compliant process validation program. Not only are they ICH guidelines but now they are also FDA guidelines. These are:

- ICH Q8—Pharmaceutical Development
  - Life cycle and risk management approach
  - Active pharmaceutical ingredient (API) and excipients
  - Container closure
  - Design space
  - Critical parameters
- ICH Q9—Quality Risk Management
  - Responsibilities
  - Risk management/integration into production
  - Risk assessment and communication
- ICH Q10—Pharmaceutical Quality System
  - Relationship with ICH Q7
  - Management responsibilities
  - Continual improvement

Food, Drug, and Cosmetic Act

SEC. 501 A drug or device shall be deemed to be adulterated

"1**(a)** (1) If it consists in whole or in part of any filthy, putrid, or decomposed substance; or **(2)**(A) if it has been prepared, packed, or held under insanitary conditions whereby it may have been contaminated with filth, or whereby it may have been rendered injurious to health; or **(B) if it is a drug and the methods used in, or the facilities or controls used for, its manufacture, processing, packing, or holding do not conform to or are not operated or administered in conformity with current good manufacturing practice to assure that such drug meets the requirements of this Act as to safety and has the identity and strength, and meets the quality and purity characteristics, which it purports or is represented to possess; or** C (3) if its container is composed, in whole or in part, of any poisonous or deleterious substance which may render the contents injurious to health; or (4) if (A) it bears or contains, for purposes of coloring only, a color additive which is . . ."

For purposes of paragraph 501(a)(2)(B), the term "current good manufacturing practice" includes the implementation of oversight and controls over the manufacture of drugs to ensure quality, including managing the risk of and establishing the safety of raw materials, materials used in the manufacturing of drugs, and finished drug products.

EXPLANATION: This has been interpreted as meaning that all drugs (veterinary or human) must meet the requirements set forth in 21 CFR 211 before they can be considered marketable. The term "current" is set forth to indicate that the expectation is that industry best practices current at the time of manufacture will be used and followed.

Title 21 Code of Federal Regulations

Sec. 211.100 Written procedures; deviations
*(a) **There shall be written procedures for production and process control designed to assure that the drug products have the identity, strength, quality, and purity they purport or are represented to possess.** Such procedures shall include all requirements in this subpart. These written procedures, including any changes, shall be drafted, reviewed, and approved by the appropriate organizational units and reviewed and approved by the quality control unit.*
*(b) **Written production and process control procedures shall be followed** in the execution of the various production and process control functions **and shall be documented at the time of performance.** Any deviation from the written procedures shall be recorded and justified.*

EXPLANATION: All functions related to the manufacture of a drug need to have a written record. This record includes the steps needed to manufacture the drug, the steps taken during the manufacture (ie, adding ingredients) and the time and person(s) performing the act. Initials or signatures indicating the completion of each step needs to be done at the time it was actually performed.

Sec. 211.22 Responsibilities of quality control unit.
*(a) There shall be a **quality control unit that shall have the responsibility and authority to approve or reject all components, drug product containers, closures, in-process materials, packaging material, labeling, and drug products, and the authority to review production records to assure that no errors have occurred or, if errors have occurred, that they have been fully investigated. The quality control unit shall be responsible for approving or rejecting drug products manufactured, processed, packed, or held under contract by another company.***

*(b) Adequate **laboratory facilities** for the testing and approval (or rejection) of components, drug product containers, closures, packaging materials, in-process materials, and drug products **shall be available to the quality control unit.***

*(c) **The quality control unit shall have the responsibility for approving or rejecting all procedures or specifications impacting on the identity, strength, quality, and purity of the drug product.***

*(d) The **responsibilities and procedures** applicable to the quality control unit **shall be in writing**; such written procedures shall be followed.*

EXPLANATION: This is one of the most critical regulations in the CFR. The Quality Unit has to approve or reject all components, documents, and investigations. They are to review the laboratory records as well.

Sec. 211.192 Production record review

All drug product production and control records, including those for packaging and labeling, *shall be* **reviewed and approved by the quality control unit to determine compliance with all established, approved written procedures before a batch is released or distributed.** *Any unexplained discrepancy (including a percentage of theoretical yield exceeding the maximum or minimum percentages established in master production and control records) or the failure of a batch or any of its components to meet any of its specifications shall be thoroughly investigated, whether or not the batch has already been distributed. The investigation shall extend to other batches of the same drug product and other drug products that may have been associated with the specific failure or discrepancy.* **A written record of the investigation shall be made and shall include the conclusions and followup**

EXPLANATION: This specifies that the Quality Unit shall conduct reviews of all production records to determine compliance with all approved written procedures.

Sec. 211.165 Testing and release for distribution.

*(a) **For each batch of drug product, there shall be appropriate laboratory determination of satisfactory conformance to final specifications for the drug product, including the identity and strength of each active ingredient,** prior to release. Where sterility and/or pyrogen testing are conducted on specific batches of short-lived radiopharmaceuticals, such batches may be released prior to completion of sterility and/or pyrogen testing, provided such testing is completed as soon as possible.*

*(b) There shall be appropriate laboratory testing, as necessary, of each batch of drug product required to be **free of objectionable microorganisms**.*

*(c) Any sampling and testing plans shall be described in **written procedures that shall include the method of sampling and the number of units per batch to be tested; such written procedure shall be followed**.*

*(d) **Acceptance criteria** for the sampling and testing conducted by the quality control unit shall be **adequate to assure** that batches of drug products **meet each appropriate specification and appropriate statistical quality control criteria** as a condition for their approval and release. The statistical quality control criteria shall include appropriate acceptance levels and/or appropriate rejection levels.*

*(e) **The accuracy, sensitivity, specificity, and reproducibility of test methods employed by the firm shall be established and documented**. Such validation and documentation may be accomplished in accordance with 211.194(a)(2).*

*(f) Drug products failing to meet established standards or specifications and any other relevant quality control criteria shall be rejected. **Reprocessing may be performed**. Prior to acceptance and use, reprocessed material must meet appropriate standards, specifications, and any other relevant criteria.*

EXPLANATION: The Quality Control laboratory needs to have written procedures just as the manufacturing area does. No Objectionable organisms[6] should be present. The laboratory equipment and test procedures require qualification and validation (except if compendial methods are followed). Statistical evaluation of the data needs to be included in determining if the product is consistent with its pre-specified release criteria.

Sec. 211.160 General requirements
*(a) **The establishment of any specifications, standards, sampling plans, test procedures, or other laboratory control mechanisms required by this subpart, including any change in such specifications, standards, sampling plans, test procedures, or other laboratory control mechanisms, shall be drafted by the appropriate organizational unit and reviewed and approved by the quality control unit. The requirements in this subpart shall be followed and shall be documented at the time of performance. Any deviation from the written specifications, standards, sampling plans, test procedures, or other laboratory control mechanisms shall be recorded and justified**.*

*(b) **Laboratory controls** shall include the establishment of **scientifically sound** and appropriate specifications, standards, sampling plans, and test procedures **designed to assure that components, drug product containers, closures, in-process materials, labeling, and drug products conform to***

appropriate standards of identity, strength, quality, and purity. *Laboratory controls shall include:*

(1) Determination of conformity to applicable written specifications for the acceptance of each lot within each shipment of components, drug product containers, closures, and labeling used in the manufacture, processing, packing, or holding of drug products. The specifications shall include a description of the sampling and testing procedures used. **Samples shall be representative and adequately identified.** *Such procedures shall also require appropriate retesting of any component, drug product container, or closure that is subject to deterioration.*

(2) **Determination of conformance** *to written specifications and a description of sampling and testing procedures* **for in-process materials**. *Such samples shall be representative and properly identified.*

(3) Determination of conformance to written descriptions of sampling procedures and appropriate specifications for drug products. Such samples shall be representative and properly identified.

(4) **The calibration of instruments, apparatus, gauges, and recording devices at suitable intervals in accordance with an established written program containing specific directions, schedules, limits for accuracy and precision**, *and provisions for remedial action in the event accuracy and/or precision limits are not met. Instruments, apparatus, gauges, and recording devices not meeting established specifications shall not be used.*

EXPLANATION: All sampling and samples taken need to be scientifically planned and the samples identified. Calibration should be performed at "suitable" intervals (industry practice is that critical instruments are to be calibrated at least every 6 months and all other instruments as needed per a written and documented program). Identity, strength, quality, and purity criteria need to be adhered to and tested against appropriate (NIST) standards. Samples need to be in containers designed for the safety and integrity of the samples (container closure testing should be performed[7]).

Sec. 211.110 Sampling and testing of in-process materials and drug products

(a) **To assure batch uniformity and integrity of drug products, written procedures shall be established and followed that describe the in-process controls, and tests, or examinations** *to be conducted on appropriate samples of in-process materials of each batch. Such control procedures shall be established to monitor the output and to validate the performance of those manufacturing processes that may be responsible for causing variability in the characteristics of in-process material and the drug product. Such control procedures shall include, but are not limited to, the following, where appropriate:*

(1) Tablet or capsule weight variation;

(2) Disintegration time;

(3) Adequacy of mixing to assure uniformity and homogeneity;

(4) Dissolution time and rate;

(5) Clarity, completeness, or pH of solutions.

(6) Bioburden testing.

(b) **Valid in-process specifications for such characteristics shall be consistent with drug product final specifications and shall be derived from previous acceptable process average and process variability estimates where possible and determined by the application of suitable statistical procedures where appropriate.** *Examination and testing of samples shall assure that the drug product and in-process material conform to specifications.*

(c) **In-process materials shall be tested for identity, strength, quality, and purity as appropriate,** *and approved or rejected by the quality control unit, during the production process, e.g., at commencement or completion of significant phases or after storage for long periods.*

(d) **Rejected in-process materials shall be identified and controlled under a quarantine system designed to prevent their use in manufacturing** *or processing operations for which they are unsuitable.*

EXPLANATION: While **211.110(a)** seems to only refer to tablets, it is intended for all pharmaceutical products (creams, ointments, semisolid) and doses as well (eg, volume, unit weight, pH, etc.). Analogous tests and conditions to those listed exist for all products. Batch uniformity needs to be verified and tested. The identity, strength, quality, and purity need to be assessed using written procedures and statistical sampling. Rejected material needs to be isolated so that it cannot be used in manufacturing (quarantined).

Sec. 211.63 Equipment design, size, and location

Equipment used in the manufacture, *processing, packing, or holding of a drug product shall be of* **appropriate design, adequate size, and suitably located** *to facilitate operations for its intended use and for its cleaning and maintenance*

EXPLANATION: Equipment needs to be suitable for its intended purpose. This includes size, type, and location within the plant. Ease of cleaning and maintenance should be considered in the design and placement of the equipment.

Sec. 211.68 Automatic, mechanical, and electronic equipment[8]

(a) **Automatic, mechanical, or electronic equipment or other types of equipment, including computers, or related systems** *that will perform a function satisfactorily, may be used in the manufacture, processing, packing, and holding of a drug product. If such equipment is so used, it* **shall be routinely calibrated, inspected, or checked according to a written program**

designed to assure proper performance. Written records of those calibration checks and inspections shall be maintained.

*(b) **Appropriate controls shall be exercised over computer or related systems to assure that changes in master production and control records or other records are instituted only by authorized personnel. Input to and output from the computer or related system of formulas or other records or data shall be checked for accuracy.** The degree and frequency of input/ output verification shall be based on the complexity and reliability of the computer or related system. **A backup file of data** entered into the computer or related system **shall be maintained** except where certain data, such as calculations performed in connection with laboratory analysis, are eliminated by computerization or other automated processes. In such instances a written record of the program shall be maintained along with appropriate validation data. **Hard copy or alternative systems**, such as duplicates, tapes, or microfilm, designed to **assure that backup data are exact and complete and that it is secure from alteration, inadvertent erasures, or loss shall be maintained.***

*(c) Such **automated equipment** used for performance of operations addressed by 211.101(c) or (d), 211.103, 211.182, or 211.188(b)(11) **can satisfy the requirements included in those sections relating to the performance of an operation by one person and checking by another person if such equipment is used in conformity with this section, and one person checks that the equipment properly performed the operation.***

EXPLANATION: Chapter 6, "Computers and Automated Systems," details the qualification and validation of computer or automated systems (this includes microchip controlled, or other control equipment). Consistency with written records needs to be established (eg, Part 11). Computer controlled or other automated systems need to have calibrations performed regularly to assure accuracy and consistency. Backup data needs to be verified for retrieveability and accuracy. If computer or other automated systems are used it is possible for the computer system to "log" the addition of materials—this would otherwise require two signatures.

Sec. 211.84 Testing and approval or rejection of components, drug product containers, and closures

(a) Each lot of components, drug product containers, and closures shall be withheld from use until the lot has been sampled, tested, or examined, as appropriate, and released for use by the quality control unit.

*(b) **Representative samples of each shipment of each lot shall be collected for testing or examination.** The **number of containers** to be **sampled**, and the amount of material to be taken from each container, shall be **based upon appropriate criteria such as statistical criteria** for component variability, confidence levels, and degree of precision desired, the past quality*

history of the supplier, and the quantity needed for analysis and reserve where required by 211.170.

(c) Samples shall be collected in accordance with the following procedures:

(1) The containers of components selected shall be cleaned when necessary in a manner to prevent introduction of contaminants into the component.

*(2) **The containers shall be opened, sampled, and resealed in a manner designed to prevent contamination of their contents and contamination of other components, drug product containers, or closures.***

(3) Sterile equipment and aseptic sampling techniques shall be used when necessary.

(4) If it is necessary to sample a component from the top, middle, and bottom of its container, such sample subdivisions shall not be composited for testing.

*(5) **Sample containers shall be identified so that the following information can be determined: name of the material sampled, the lot number, the container from which the sample was taken, the date on which the sample was taken, and the name of the person who collected the sample.***

*(6) **Containers** from which samples have been taken shall be **marked to show that samples have been removed** from them.*

(d) Samples shall be examined and tested as follows:

*(1) **At least one test shall be conducted to verify the identity** of each component of a drug product. Specific identity tests, if they exist, shall be used.*

(2) Each component shall be tested for conformity with all appropriate written specifications for purity, strength, and quality. In lieu of such testing by the manufacturer, a report of analysis may be accepted from the supplier of a component, provided that at least one specific identity test is conducted on such component by the manufacturer, and provided that the manufacturer establishes the reliability of the supplier's analyses through appropriate validation of the supplier's test results at appropriate intervals.

*(3) **Containers and closures shall be tested for conformity with all appropriate written specifications.** In lieu of such testing by the manufacturer, a certificate of testing may be accepted from the supplier, provided that at least a visual identification is conducted on such containers/closures by the manufacturer and provided that the manufacturer establishes the reliability of the supplier's test results through appropriate validation of the supplier's test results at appropriate intervals.*

(4) When appropriate, components shall be microscopically examined.

(5) Each lot of a component, drug product container, or closure that is liable to contamination with filth, insect infestation, or other extraneous adulterant shall be examined against established specifications for such contamination.

(6) Each lot of a component, drug product container, or closure with potential for microbiological contamination that is objectionable in view of its intended use shall be subjected to microbiological tests before use.

(e) Any lot of components, drug product containers, or closures that meets the appropriate written specifications of identity, strength, quality, and purity and related tests under paragraph (d) of this section may be approved and released for use. Any lot of such material that does not meet such specifications shall be rejected.

EXPLANATION: Containers used for sampling need to be clean and free of contaminants that will interfere with testing of the sample. The containers need to be clearly identified. Sampling of raw material should be done in a way so as to not introduce contaminants. Statistical sampling is to be employed so as to obtain a true representative sample.

Sec. 211.42 Design and construction features

*(a) Any **building** or buildings used in the manufacture, processing, packing, or holding of a drug product shall be of **suitable size, construction and location to facilitate cleaning, maintenance, and proper operations**.*

*(b) Any such building shall have **adequate space for the orderly placement of equipment and materials to prevent mixups** between different components, drug product containers, closures, labeling, in-process materials, or drug products, and to prevent contamination. The flow of components, drug product containers, closures, labeling, in-process materials, and drug products through the building or buildings shall be designed to prevent contamination.*

(c) Operations shall be performed within specifically defined areas of adequate size. There shall be separate or defined areas or such other control systems for the firm's operations as are necessary to prevent contamination or mixups during the course of the following procedures:

(1) Receipt, identification, storage, and withholding from use of components, drug product containers, closures, and labeling, pending the appropriate sampling, testing, or examination by the quality control unit before release for manufacturing or packaging;

(2) Holding rejected components, drug product containers, closures, and labeling before disposition;

(3) Storage of released components, drug product containers, closures, and labeling;

(4) Storage of in-process materials;

(5) Manufacturing and processing operations;

(6) Packaging and labeling operations;

(7) Quarantine storage before release of drug products;

(8) Storage of drug products after release;

(9) Control and laboratory operations;

(10) Aseptic processing, which includes as appropriate:

(i) Floors, walls, and ceilings of smooth, hard surfaces that are easily cleanable;

(ii) Temperature and humidity controls;

(iii) An air supply filtered through high-efficiency particulate air filters under positive pressure, regardless of whether flow is laminar or nonlaminar;

(iv) A system for monitoring environmental conditions;

(v) A system for cleaning and disinfecting the room and equipment to produce aseptic conditions;

(vi) A system for maintaining any equipment used to control the aseptic conditions.
(d) Operations relating to the manufacture, processing, and packing of penicillin shall be performed in facilities separate from those used for other drug products for human use.

EXPLANATION: Pharmaceutical facilities need to be of sufficient size and location so as to facilitate the manufacturing process. Care needs to be taken to assure that there is sufficient room for all equipment for all operations. Prevention of mix-ups is very important, not only on the final product but throughout the entire operation (all components, materials, etc.)

Sec. 211.44 Lighting.
Adequate lighting shall be provided in all areas.

EXPLANATION: The amount of light in each work area needs to be predicated on the type of work being performed.

Sec. 211.46 Ventilation, air filtration, air heating and cooling[9]
(a) Adequate ventilation shall be provided.
(b) Equipment for adequate control over air pressure, micro-organisms, dust, humidity, and temperature shall be provided when appropriate for the manufacture, processing, packing, or holding of a drug product.
*(c) Air filtration systems, including prefilters and particulate matter air filters, shall be used when appropriate on air supplies to production areas. If air is recirculated to production areas, **measures shall be taken to control recirculation of dust from production**. In areas where air contamination occurs during production, there shall be adequate exhaust systems or other systems adequate to control contaminants.*
*(d) **Air-handling systems for the manufacture, processing, and packing of penicillin shall be completely separate from those for other drug products for human use.***

EXPLANATION: The quality of the air in the facility is predicated upon the exposure of the product to possible contamination.

Sec. 211.48 Plumbing.
*(a) **Potable water shall be supplied under continuous positive pressure** in a plumbing system free of defects that could contribute contamination to any drug product. Potable water shall meet the standards prescribed in the Environmental Protection Agency's Primary Drinking Water Regulations set forth in 40 CFR part 141. Water not meeting such standards shall not be permitted in the potable water system.*
(b) Drains shall be of adequate size and, where connected directly to a sewer, shall be provided with an air break or other mechanical device to prevent back-siphonage.

EXPLANATION: Potable water (drinking water quality) is required as the starting point for water to be used in production. Water reports from the source (municipal utility) as well as reports taken for purified water or water for injection are often included in the annual product report.

Sec. 211.186 Master production and control records

(a) To assure uniformity from batch to batch, master production and control records for **each drug product, including each batch size thereof, shall be prepared, dated, and signed (full signature, handwritten) by one person and independently checked, dated, and signed by a second person**. The preparation of master production and control records shall be described in a written procedure and such written procedure shall be followed.

(b) Master production and control records shall include:

(1) The **name and strength of the product** and a description of the dosage form;

(2) The **name and weight or measure of each active ingredient** per dosage unit or per unit of weight or measure of the drug product, and a statement of the total weight or measure of any dosage unit;

(3) A **complete list of components** designated by names or codes sufficiently specific to indicate any special quality characteristic;

(4) An **accurate statement of the weight or measure of each component**, using the same weight system (metric, avoirdupois, or apothecary) for each component. **Reasonable variations may be permitted**, however, in the amount of components necessary for the preparation in the dosage form, pro-vided they are justified in the master production and control records;

(5) **A statement concerning any calculated excess of component**;

(6) A statement of **theoretical weight** or measure at appropriate phases of processing;

(7) A statement of **theoretical yield**, including the maximum and minimum percentages of theoretical yield beyond which investigation according to 211.192 is required;

(8) A description of the drug product containers, closures, and packaging materials, including a specimen or **copy of each label** and all other labeling signed and dated by the person or persons responsible for approval of such labeling;

(9) **Complete manufacturing and control instructions, sampling and testing procedures, specifications, special notations, and precautions to be followed.**

EXPLANATION: Master Batch Records need to list: Name and strength of the product; weight of each API with a total unit weight; complete list of all components with weights; calculated theoretical yield and weights; a copy of each label; complete manufacturing instructions.

Sec. 211.188 Batch production and control records

Batch production and control records shall be prepared for each batch of drug product produced and **shall include complete information relating to the production and control of each batch.** These records shall include:

(a) An **accurate reproduction of the appropriate master production or control record, checked for accuracy, dated, and signed;**

(b) **Documentation that each significant step** in the manufacture, processing, packing, or holding of the batch **was accomplished,** including:

(1) Dates;

(2) **Identity of individual major equipment and lines used;**

(3) **Specific identification of each batch of component** or in-process material used;

(4) **Weights and measures of components used in the course of processing;**

(5) **In-process and laboratory control results;**

(6) **Inspection of the packaging and labeling area before and after use;**

(7) A statement of **the actual yield** and a statement of the **percentage of theoretical yield** at appropriate phases of processing;

(8) **Complete labeling control records,** including specimens or copies of all labeling used;

(9) **Description of drug product containers and closures;**

(10) Any **sampling performed;**

(11) **Identification of the persons performing and directly supervising or checking each significant step in the operation, or if a significant step in the operation is performed by automated equipment under 211.68, the identification of the person checking the significant step performed by the automated equipment.**

(12) **Any investigation** made according to 211.192.

(13) Results of examinations made in accordance with 211.134.

EXPLANATION: Similar requirements as to the Master Batch Record and must be an exact copy. The production batch record needs to have the following information: Identity of all components used; actual weights of all components; sampling results; second review and signature of significant steps (can be a computer verification); percentage of theoretical yield; results of any investigations.

Sec. 211.180 General requirements

(a) **Any production, control, or distribution record** that is required to be maintained in compliance with this part and is specifically associated with a batch of a drug product **shall be retained for at least 1 year after the expiration date of the batch** or, in the case of certain OTC drug products lacking expiration dating because they meet the criteria for exemption under 211.137, 3 years after distribution of the batch.

(b) **Records shall be maintained for all components, drug product containers, closures, and labeling for at least 1 year after the expiration**

date or, in the case of certain OTC drug products lacking expiration dating because they meet the criteria for exemption under 211.137, 3 years after distribution of the last lot of drug product incorporating the component or using the container, closure, or labeling.

(c) **All records** required under this part, or copies of such records, **shall be readily available for authorized inspection during the retention period** at the establishment where the activities described in such records occurred. These records or copies thereof shall be subject to photocopying or other means of reproduction as part of such inspection. Records that can be immediately retrieved from another location by computer or other electronic means shall be considered as meeting the requirements of this paragraph.

(d) **Records required under this part may be retained either as original records or as true copies such as photocopies, microfilm, microfiche, or other accurate reproductions of the original records.** Where reduction techniques, such as microfilming, are used, suitable reader and photocopying equipment shall be readily available.

(e) **Written records** required by this part shall be maintained so that data therein can be used for **evaluating, at least annually,** the quality standards of each drug product to determine the need for changes in drug product specifications or manufacturing or control procedures. Written procedures shall be established and followed for such evaluations and shall include provisions for:

(1) **A review of a representative number of batches, whether approved or rejected, and, where applicable, records associated with the batch.**

(2) **A review of complaints, recalls, returned or salvaged drug products, and investigations conducted under 211.192 for each drug product.**

(f) Procedures shall be established to assure that the **responsible officials of the firm,** if they are not personally involved in or immediately aware of such actions, **are notified in writing of any investigations** conducted under 211.198, 211.204, or 211.208 of these regulations, any recalls, reports of inspectional observations issued by the Food and Drug Administration, or any regulatory actions relating to good manufacturing practices brought by the Food and Drug Administration.

EXPLANATION: This regulation sets forth the need to retain all product records for at least 1 year after the expiration date of the product. The records need to be reviewed annually. Also, a responsible person in the firm needs to be notified of all investigations, recalls, etc.

FDA—Compliance Program Guidance (CPG)

CPG 7356.02—API Process Inspection

This covers the FDA's expectations during an API inspection. It covers the plant Quality Systems, Facilities and Equipment, Material systems, Productions systems, Packaging and labeling, and Laboratory control systems. This guide can be used in conjunction with the ICH guideline for the GMP regulations for APIs.

CPG 490.100—Process Validation Requirements for Drug Products and APIs Subject to Pre-Market Approval

This document covers both sterile and nonsterile products. Conformation batches do not need to be completed for the NDA to be approved. However, at least one conformation batch should be successful prior to distribution. It goes on to discuss pre- and postapproval inspections.

CPG 7132a.07—Computerized Drug Processing; Input/Output Checking

All of these documents are related to computer systems used in the pharmaceutical environment. Firms have flexibility on the verification timing and extent of data analysis of Input/Output (I/O) information.

CPG 7132a.08—Computerized Drug Processing: Identification of "Persons" on Batch Production and Control Records

Validation of the computer system is required when using it as a "Person" during production. It also requires that 21 CFR 211.188(b)(11) be followed.

CPG 7132a.11—Computerized Drug Processing; CGMP Applicability to Hardware and Software

Where a computer is being used in a GMP function the hardware is regarded as equipment and the application software is regarded as records.

CPG 7132a.15—Computerized Drug Processing; Source Code for Process Control Application Programs

Source code and supporting documentation needs to be reviewed and approved prior to its use. The review should include all operation conditions and requirements. 21 CFR 211 100, 180, 186 should be adhered to for the data and all records. The source code is also considered to be part of the Master Batch Record.

American Society for Testing and Materials (ASTM)

E 2500-07—Standard Guide for Specification, Design, and Verification of Pharmaceutical and Biopharmaceutical Manufacturing Systems and Equipment

This guide is the basis for the QbD approach to pharmaceutical manufacturing. It uses ICH Q9 for its risk management and ICH Q8 for development. It details Good Engineering Practice, design reviews, and change management. It also separates out a verification program that should be used for equipment and facilities.

E 2810-11—Standard Practice for Demonstrating Capability to Comply with the Test for Uniformity of Dosage Units

This document details how to determine the acceptance criteria and statistical samples necessary to be assured of compliance to content uniformity requirements. It provides a methodology to generate an acceptance limit table.

ASTM-E2474—Standard Practice for Pharmaceutical Process Design Utilizing Process Analytical Technology

This covers pharmaceutical process design utilizing process analytical technology, which is integral to process development as well as postdevelopment process optimization. It is focused on practical implementation and experimental development of process understanding. The principles in this practice are applicable to both drug substance and drug product processes.

NOTES

1. ASTM E 2500-07; Standard Guide for Specification, Design, and Verification of Pharmaceutical and Biopharmaceutical Manufacturing Systems and Equipment; Jun. 2007.

2. Guidance for Industry Process Validation: General Principles and Practices, FDA, Jan. 2011.

3. Guidance for Industry: Q7A Good Manufacturing Practice Guidance for Active Pharmaceutical Ingredients; FDA, Aug. 2001.

4. Guide to the Inspections Validation of Cleaning Processes; FDA Jul. 1993.

5. ICH is formed by the United States, European Union, and Japan and is binding on each of these "countries" so as to facilitate inspections respectively.

6. United States Pharmacopeia; Microbiological Examination of Non-Sterile Products: Microbial Enumeration Tests <61>; and Microbiological Examination of Non-Sterile Products: Tests for Specified Microorganisms <62>; United States Pharmacopeial Convention, Inc.

7. Guidance for Industry: Container Closure Systems for Packaging Human Drugs and Biologics; FDA, May. 1999.

8. Refer to Title 21 Code of Federal Regulations Part 11; 2015.

9. NOTE: If the product is penicillin or related products (eg, cephalosporins) the air and facility must be isolated to prevent even the smallest cross-over due to the possible highly allergic status of this class of drug.

CHAPTER 3

The Validation Life Cycle and Change Control

LIFE CYCLE APPROACH

Until the 2011 US Food and Drug Administration (FDA) guideline on process validation was released, companies defaulted to making three batches in order to complete their process validation. With the release of the 2011[1] guideline the emphasis changed to a risk-based approach, and the risk relies on the process life cycle. The risk referred to here is the chance of an error during production adversely affecting a patient. A life cycle[2] means that each step of the process relies on the step before and the step after. While other parts of the process, for example, cleaning, aseptic processes, computer systems, have their own "life cycles" approach, this book is primarily dedicated to the process validation life cycle itself. The Current Good Manufacturing Practices (CGMPs) are all of 21 CFR Part 211, however, only certain aspects of these as they pertain to process validation will be discussed. Additional guidelines dealing with other topics related to process validation such as the Aseptic Processing[3] and Cleaning Validation[4] Guidelines are available. Appendix B provides a short list of some additional guidelines that are helpful when getting ready to start a process validation program. The FDA web site (http://www.fda.gov) has a full listing of guidelines and other helpful documents to assist in meeting all FDA compliance requirements.

The Code of Federal Regulations[5] (CFR) sets the regulations for all Good Manufacturing Practice (GMP) activities (see Chapter 2: A Brief Review of the Regulations). As previously addressed in Chapter 1, "Introduction to Process Validation," there are now three major stages to a complete process validation program. However, process validation does not start, or end, with these three stages.

By following the guidelines the pharmaceutical manufacturer can make the necessary adjustments to the process so as to maintain proper records and achieve reproducible results and full compliance with the current GMP regulations. Fig. 3.1[6] shows the process validation life cycle adopted from a presentation by the FDA.[7] This fits into the

How to Validate a Pharmaceutical Process. DOI: http://dx.doi.org/10.1016/B978-0-12-804148-2.00003-2

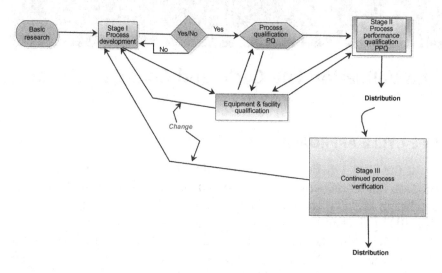

Figure 3.1 Process validation life cycle. Source: Modified from G. McNally, FDA.[6]

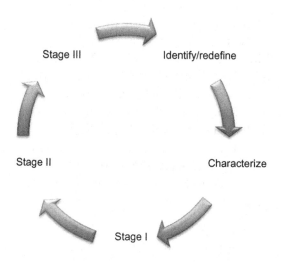

Figure 3.2 Simple life cycle approach.

general validation life cycle as seen in Fig. 3.2. From this diagram, it should be clear that the entire project, from initial conception through implementation of the final production is part of the CGMP compliance program. Note that Fig. 3.1 just addresses the process validation portion.

One aspect that is often left out of the validation life cycle is the need for staff training in each area. Each part of the cycle requires its own level of training. All employees need training on at least a basic level of CGMPs as well as more specific training for their jobs. The training program and all employees should stay current with the CGMPs, as well as the use, maintenance, cleaning, and operation of all process equipment. The validation group also needs training and experience in the use of the test instruments, sample selection and handling, protocol development, execution, and record keeping (ie, Good Documentation Practices).

The technology transfer program, that is, moving the process from the pilot plant to production, also calls for a high degree of training by the "sending" team to the "receiving" team.[8] All of this must fall under the change control program.

THE ROLE OF CHANGE CONTROL

The change control program is the mainstay of maintaining a compliant state of the process or operation. It is used in every aspect of the process, from equipment changes through process parameter changes. Since the compliance program is ongoing, all modifications, regardless of how small, must be done under a formal change control program.

The purpose of a change control program is to have a written record of any, and all, changes that occur to the equipment, process, or supporting documentation, including computer software and/or Programmable Logic Controller (PLC) code. An important outcome of a working change control program is that all documents related to the changed item(s) are updated and reapproved if necessary. These documents include the User Requirements (URS), Functional Requirements (FRS), Design Specifications (DS), Traceability Matrix (TM), Standard Operation Procedures (SOP), and other life cycle validation documents.

As stated, change control is a key element of the production process. The FDA expects that all processes undergo "continuous improvement." In order to do this, changes have to be made to the process. These changes can, and often do, include changes in equipment, operating conditions, or even the location of the equipment to improve product flow.

The first question often asked is "When does change control start?" Change control starts when GMPs begin. The program should be put into place before the qualification starts. It becomes active upon completion of the commissioning of the equipment, since any change in the unit from that time will impact its GMP readiness. That is, at the very first entry into an equipment qualification protocol. Thus, change control does not apply to basic research operations. The researcher is free to use any chemicals, equipment, or procedural steps while they are searching for the most effective pharmaceutical agent.

Once the Installation Qualification (IQ) protocol execution is started for a piece of equipment you need to make changes via the change control program. In order to make any change in a process after the equipment has been qualified and the process validated a change control form needs to be completed. The reason for this is simple; the equipment was designed in a specific manner to perform a specific function so any change or deviation from the "expected" needs to be documented.

The above is not meant to exclude recording changes made during commissioning. While these changes or fixes are not usually under the change control program, any changes made during commissioning also need to be recorded. These changes will then be reflected in the qualification protocols (eg, IQ or Operational Qualification, OQ). By definition then, changes made during commissioning (getting the equipment ready for use) are not generally considered as part of the change control process. In fact, one usually keeps these changes separate so that time is not lost getting the equipment ready for use. Whether to keep commissioning under the change control program is a decision of the Quality Unit of the company.

In addition to any changes made during commissioning or qualification, change control also applies during production. Anyone can make a request for a change to the equipment or process. For example, this could include equipment improvements, process improvements, or flow improvements. Prior to making any changes, either during qualification or during production, a change request form needs to be completed. In this form the change to be made is identified and the reason clearly defined. An example of a simple Change Control form can be seen in Appendix C. This then is forwarded to several departments for review and approvals as indicated:

- Supervisor—needs to review and approve the requested change
- Engineering/Maintenance—reviews for engineering concerns, possibility of the change from the equipment perspective
- Validation—reviews the request for testing needed to maintain or improve GMP compliance

- Management—reviews for cost-effectiveness
- Quality/Regulatory—reviews for compliance to company standards and FDA (or foreign regulatory agency) requirements

TYPES OF CHANGES[9]

Now that the reason for recording changes has been established let's review the classifications of changes used in the pharmaceutical industry. These are classified as:

- Major
- Minor
- Required or Emergency
- Local/Deferred

These can be summarized in the flowcharts shown in Figs. 3.3 and 3.4. Let us take a brief look at each type. The FDA has a guideline specifying what should be reported to them and when it should be reported.[9]

A major change requires that the FDA be notified, and approval obtained, prior to implementing the change. This type of change occurs when a piece of process equipment is changed (eg, changing blender types or designs, change of process parameters replacement of a "ribbon" blender with a "V" blender). Major changes are also those changes that may occur due to a change in the vendor for the active ingredient (API). The reason for this is that changing the API vendor or one type of process equipment for another, even if the function and capacity are the same, could result in a change in a Critical Quality Attribute (CQA) of the product; thus, jeopardizing the compliant state of the entire process.

A minor change can be reported in the Annual Product Report (APR). These changes are usually due to a continuous improvement program (eg, changing warehouse location). In any case, it is up to the Quality Unit (eg, QA) and the regulatory affairs groups to determine when and how the FDA should be notified of the change.

A required change is just as the name implies. The FDA or other regulatory agency requires that a change in the equipment or process be made (eg, need to add a check weigher to the line due to a need to weigh each container to assure proper addition of ingredients).

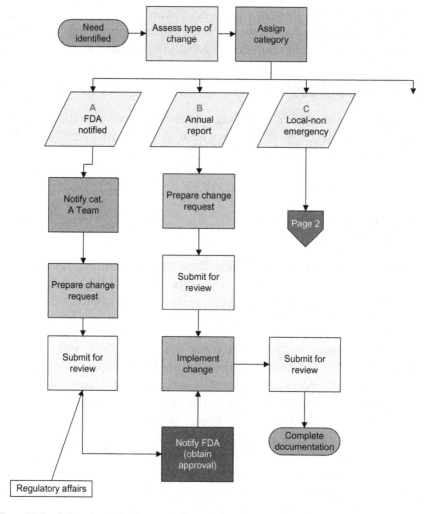

Figure 3.3 Simple flow chart of the change control process. Source: Informa Healthcare.

Another example is emergency changes that can occur and need to be addressed immediately. Those changes mandated by any of the regulatory agencies should be made as quickly as possible and documented as to what and how the change was made. Emergency changes occur at times when least expected. Following a complete and comprehensive preventative maintenance program can minimize the need for these changes. In an emergency it is not usually necessary to prepare and file the document for change control at the time of the emergency. In all cases, it is always preferable for the change to be a "like-for-like" item. If this is not possible QA must formally authorize the change and the

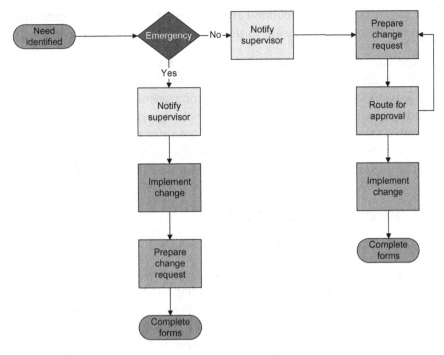

Figure 3.4 Continuation of the change control flow. Source: Informa Healthcare.

product will need to have further tested. The emergency must be recti-fied first and then the paperwork **MUST** be submitted. This allows the QA department to make a determination about the status of the batch if one was involved. Most companies allow 24 h or the next business day from the emergency before filing the papers. In these situations additional product testing, stability studies, etc. may be ordered.

An example of a local change is one in which a change is needed in an SOP or other GMP document. Changes to SOPs, which are related to the process, are also reported in the APR. The local type is by far the most common of all changes, that is, any change that takes place in an SOP, or other GMP document related to the operation or use of manufacturing equipment, must be controlled and documented (and retraining performed) under the change control program. This includes even minor corrections such as a spelling error in an SOP. Other exam-ples of local changes may be renaming or renumbering the SOPs, repla-cing a label on a piece of equipment or improvements related to safety.

A deferred change (not very common) are minor changes to a system that might be identified and then placed on hold until a more convenient time for execution, or a required change is made and then implemented. This allows for their inclusion in the change evaluation assessment.

Applying the change control program is necessary from the start of GMPs. That is, from the signing of the first equipment qualification protocol. Once the protocol is signed, components cannot be changed or adjustments made without using the change control program. It is advisable to get the equipment ready for use prior to beginning the qualification. This is the purpose of the commissioning phase of the project (as discussed in Chapter 5: Basic Equipment and Utility Qualification).

THE CHANGE CONTROL PROCESS[10]

A typical approach to change control is outlined as follows:

1. A change is thought to be necessary (eg, a line operator thinks that changing a manual valve to any automatic valve will not only make his/her job easier but also makes the product more consistent as it will not be dependent on an operator's decision).
2. The operator writes up his idea and submits it to his/her supervisor.
3. The supervisor decides whether it is a worthwhile idea and sends it to his/her supervisor or to the line manager.
4. The line manager reviews it and sends it to engineering.
5. Engineering reviews it and sends it to QA/regulatory/validation.
6. QA (regulatory and/or validation) approves and sends it to upper management. The GMP status of the requested change is evaluated. If there is an apparent impact of the GMP or compliance status of the requested change it still may be approved, but further consideration is needed (how it can be brought into compliance again).
7. Management reviews and finally approves or rejects. If the change request is approved, then the affected departments will be notified. Usually this means engineering, validation, QA, and the requesting group.

However, at any point in the review process any of the reviewing parties can stop the idea for any reason: cost, time, value, or how it will affect the GMP status of the equipment or the process (ie, the line may have to be requalified or revalidated. This general outline is shown in Figs. 3.3 and 3.4. The flowchart represented here is broken into the major areas as discussed above, but the basic review cycle is the same. Thus, the following departments/groups are usually involved in the change control: Operations, Engineering/Maintenance, Validation, Quality, Management (at different levels based on change scope and cost). Other departments may also become involved such as the Regulatory Affairs and Safety departments.

A change control form has the following information[10] (also seen in Appendix C is an abbreviated Change Control form):

Part 1: Origination
1. Name of originating person
2. Date requested
3. Date needed
4. Reason for request
5. Justification (as necessary)
6. Supervisors' approval

Part 2: Other Departments and Management (last)
1. Date received
2. Reviewer
3. Disposition
4. Reason for disposition
5. Date sent back or forwarded

Part 3: Validation
1. Date received
2. Reviewer
3. Compliance Impact Assessment
4. Disposition
5. Date forwarded or rejected

Part 4: To File
1. Date received

When supporting a change control request, all necessary engineering, validation, and production information must either be attached, or its location referenced, for easy retrieval and review.

NOTES

1. Guidance for Industry Process Validation: General Principles and Practices, FDA, Jan. 2011.

2. Pluta, P.: FDA Life Cycle Approach to Process Validation—What, Why, and How. J. Validation Technology Spring, 51–61; 2011.

3. Guidance for Industry: Sterile Drug Products Produced by Aseptic Processing—Current Good Manufacturing Practice; FDA, Sep. 2004.

4. Guide to the Inspections Validation of Cleaning Processes; FDA Jul. 1993.

5. Title 21 Code of Federal Regulations Parts 210 and 211, 2015.

6. Process Validation A Life Cycle Approach; Grace McNally; FDA May 2011 slide presentation on www.FDA.gov

7. Ibid.

8. Sending team—those responsible for the current operation and instrumental in training and transferring their knowledge to the receiving team.

9. Guidance for Industry: CMC Postapproval Manufacturing Changes to be Documented in Annual Reports; FDA—Mar. 2014.

10. Ostrove, S.: Qualification and Change Control. In: Validation of Pharmaceutical Processes, 3rd Ed; Editors: Agalloco, J., Carlton, F. New York: Informa Healthcare USA, Inc., 2008, pp. 129–145.

Stage I—Process Development

Getting Started

BEFORE IT ALL STARTS

As presented in Chapter 1, "Introduction to Process Validation" process validation (PV) is a program that requires the interaction of several groups, not just one individual. Thus, the first thing that needs to be addressed is the organization and assembly of the necessary groups to plan the validation effort (Fig. 4.1). The actual plan for the validation program is documented in the Validation Master Plan (VMP). This document usually requires several months to prepare and involves the input from many different groups within the manufacturing site. Some of the main groups or departments that should be tapped for input are:

- Analytical Lab
- Engineering/Maintenance
- Metrology
- Operations
- Quality
- Regulatory Affairs
- Research & Development
- Validation

Others may be involved for parts of the planning, for example, Health & Safety, Document Control, IT, etc., since almost every department will have some input into the program. The announcement of the project should be widely distributed and meetings publicized to

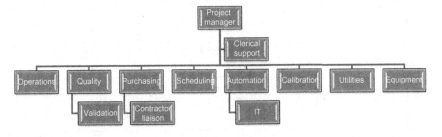

Figure 4.1 Organization chart for a process validation project.

How to Validate a Pharmaceutical Process. DOI: http://dx.doi.org/10.1016/B978-0-12-804148-2.00004-4

allow input from all sources. A project manager or coordinator will integrate all aspects of the project and increase the likelihood that the project will run smoothly. The size of the facility, the types of products, and the experience of the staff (training) will have major impacts on the execution of the project.

Each department should provide the input necessary based on their expertise or needs. For example, the operations group will know how the equipment will be used during actual commercial production. They are the ones who will be providing the user requirements to the engineering group. The engineers will then develop the functional requirements and, subsequently, the design requirements. The functional requirements are those that set the way the equipment will operate and thus be able to perform their user requirements. The design requirements are those that are used to actually make the unit work, that includes the programming, the utility requirements, as well as all the process specifications. After the design is complete the request is sent to the purchasing department who will then request bids (with specifications) from vendors who can provide the unit of choice. Fig. 4.2 shows a general approach to a project that starts with the pharmaceutical company and moves through validation consultants and to the vendor.

Example

A user requirement can be the need for a blender that needs to hold 500 kg of material. The functional requirement then would specify that the unit be able to hold 750–1000 kg (Note: The unit should normally hold 50–100% more than required. This also goes for sizing the motors, etc. so as to keep the duty cycle in an effective range and extend the life of

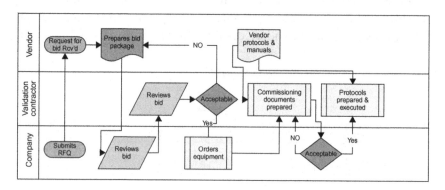

Figure 4.2 General project flow.

the equipment) of material, thus it would need to be XX by XX Ft^2. This information would then be given to the engineering group who would put the unit together allowing sufficient rotation space (Note: All equipment should be installed allowing sufficient room on all sides to service the unit). Fig. 4.3 shows a blender installation allowing sufficient room for rotation and maintenance. The need for access to all sides of the equipment applies to the utilities as well as the process equipment. In another approach, the user requirements may be turned over to the purchasing department who will then order a unit from a vendor that can provide the necessary requirements. The engineering department and the operations department prior to actually placing the order should check this request. This is also known as bid verification or bid review, which is a very important step that is often omitted due to project time constraints.

GETTING STARTED (AFTER THE EQUIPMENT SPECIFICATIONS)

Process validation cannot begin when the first commercial size batch is produced. It must start much earlier. In reality, process validation begins in the basic research stage. While basic research itself is not under Good Manufacturing Practices (GMPs), the results that are obtained there are critical to successfully completing the PV process.

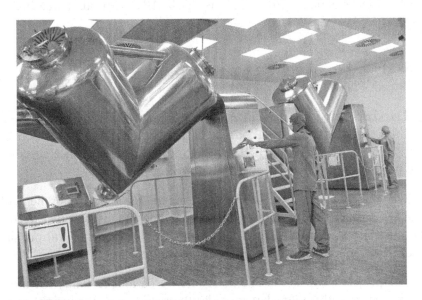

Figure 4.3 Example of a V Blender. Source: Dmitry Kalinovsky/Shutterstock.

There is a lot of information that needs to be collected and organized prior to starting an effective process validation program. There are four major categories of documents that are needed for any successful process validation project. These are:

- VMP
- Standard Operating Procedures (SOPs)
- Quality Programs (as standards)
- Protocols—(Commissioning, Equipment and Utility Qualifications, Process Performance Qualification)

Table 4.1 is a "wish list" of recommended documents and information that one should try to collect prior to starting the process validation. Many of these documents and drawings are critical to preparing the VMP. Others are needed for the protocols or SOPs. Be aware that each project is unique and not all documents are needed for every project. For example, the facility layout should also be available for the VMP so as to be able to show the paths that the materials and people will take in producing the product(s).

THE VALIDATION MASTER PLAN

As previously stated, before beginning any validation program there needs to be a plan. In this case it is the VMP. There are three major types of VMPs:

- Corporate Plan
- Site Plan
- Project Plan

The corporate plan is used to outline the general functions, responsibilities, products, and methods to be used during the production of any pharmaceutical product. It is a high level document since specifics will be provided in the site plan or the project plan.

The site master plan provides more detail for the development of projects at each site (assuming more than one manufacturing site for the company). However, it is also useful for a single operation site since it will guide the project plans in the future.

The project VMP is the one most often used and certainly the most referenced. It is this plan that provides the reader with the insight as to what is included in the project, how it will be accomplished, and by

Table 4.1 Wish List

Reports

Development

Balance (eg, HVAC)

Cleaning

Passivation

Vendor tests—FAT/SAT

Weld

Drawings

PFD

P&ID

Vendor

Isometrics (WFI systems only)

Equipment layout

Air flow

People flow

Material flow

  Material

    In process

    Raw materials

    Waste material

Manuals

Cleaning

Operation

Preventive maintenance

SOPs

Backup

Calibration

Change control

Cleaning

Emergency

Sampling

Operation

Preventive maintenance

Training

Storage/warehousing

  In process

  Finished

(*Continued*)

Table 4.1 (Continued)
Specifications
Engineering design
Functional requirement specifications (FRS)
Operating ranges
Critical process parameters
Critical quality Attributes
User requirements (URS)
Other Documents
Standards
Computer/systems
Ladder logic
Source code
Batch records
List of critical/noncritical instruments
Contractor certifications
Personnel qualifications
Equipment certifications
Logs
Equipment use
Cleaning

whom and when the tasks will be completed. It serves to guide and at the end assure that the validation effort is complete.

While the project VMP is a guide not only for those involved in the project, it is also a guide for corporate management and the regulatory agencies. Thus, it is important to include not only the equipment to be qualified and a basic approach as to how that is to be done, but also the processes to be validated and the rationale as to why it is being validated in this manner (Note: there are always several approaches that can be taken to validate a process; selecting the path that is defendable, scientifically sound, and risk-based is what is needed).

Having a complete equipment list is essential. All process and support equipment needs to be identified and described in the VMP. Their function in the process and some general information as to how they will be qualified is part of a good master plan. One suggestion is to attach the equipment list to the appendix of the VMP. Placing it there will allow the manufacturer to keep the equipment list updated without having to send the VMP around for review and signatures each time the equipment is updated (this is especially important for contract manufacturers who are always changing equipment in and out based on the needs of their clients).

One section of the VMP that should always be included is a time line for the project. This is intended to help not only the project team keep to a schedule, but it is also for the use of the regulatory agencies to determine the thought and commitment to the project. Since the VMP is a living document, it would be expected that the time line be continually updated as the project progresses. This is not always feasible. Thus, one suggestion is to note on the time line that it was prepared on a particular date and will be updated upon re-review of the VMP or sooner if necessary. This section or time line also can be part of the appendix of the document so it can be updated as necessary without sending the entire VMP around again for review and approval. Tables 4.2 and 4.3 list a generic table of contents for a project VMP. The VMP, like all GMP documents, should have a scheduled review cycle. The review period varies from company to company, but once it is set it needs to be adhered to completely.

What constitutes a good VMP? One that is easy to read, easy to follow (allowing the reader to understand how the product will flow

Table 4.2 VMP Table of Contents

- Approvals
- Scope
- Responsibilities/personnel
- Facility description
- Process description
- Validation approach
- Utility description
- Equipment description
- Process description
  - Process validation approach
- Documents
  - SOPs
  - Protocol list
  - Equipment history file
- Ancillary validation programs
  - Cleaning
  - Analytical methods
  - Preventive maintenance
  - Change control
  - Training
  - Pest control
- Appendix
  - Sample SOPs
  - Sample protocol form

Table 4.3 Diagrams to Include in the VMP

- Flow diagrams
  - Material
  - Air
  - People
  - Process
- Equipment layout

through the facility without cross-contamination or mix-ups) and provides sufficient information about the facility design, the product(s) to be manufactured, and the supporting systems that are in place to assure compliance with the Current Good Manufacturing Practices (CGMPs).

STANDARD OPERATING PROCEDURES (SOPs) PREPARATION

In the preparation of SOPs there are often higher levels of documents that control the functionality of the various systems and operations. At a corporate level there are the corporate policies. These are general documents that set a goal for all plant or corporate functions. Below these policies are the standards. These are usually prepared at the site level so that each facility (assuming more than one site) applies the policies to their particular products or environmental conditions. From these standards the SOPs are prepared. SOPs are documents that inform the process operators, maintenance staff, and others about what has to be done and how it is to be done. For example, there should be an SOP for how to prepare an SOP, or an SOP on how to execute a process validation protocol. In some cases the SOPs are further subdivided into work orders which provide more specific information, for example, how to disassemble a particular process piece of equipment for cleaning.

An SOP should be easy to follow and be specific for the particular function. All documents (SOPs, protocols, etc.) should be easy to follow, as this is key to having the employees meet full compliance. While the format is not a GMP item, the content is. Appendix A provides a simple example of an SOP for preparing a VMP.

There should be an SOP to explain how to operate of each piece of equipment as well as its maintenance and cleaning procedures. Other SOPs that are needed are emergency plans, backup of data, sampling, etc. Some of these SOPs become very long, thus the work orders providing the detail needed to disassemble or reassemble a unit, are important.

QUALITY PROGRAMS

The Quality Program approach should be used for all CGMP activities. The FDA and the ICH have guidelines[1,2] regarding this approach (see Appendix C). The Quality Programs are major sets of plans that are needed for a successful process validation program. Table 4.4 lists some of the more common Quality Programs needed for a well-rounded process validation.

These programs must be kept up to date with current GMPs as well as current corporate policies. These programs are the responsibility of the manager of the departments who then must assure that the staff adheres to the programs and are fully trained on them as well as on all SOP required for their job function. The Quality Programs are more of a high level approach to maintaining CGMP status throughout the operation.

The Quality System program is a major part of the FDAs inspections system—Quality System Inspection Technique.[3] With this the FDA holds management responsible for compliance.

TRAINING

A training program is one of the core quality programs and is required for all personnel working in a pharmaceutical facility. This requirement can be found in 21 CFR 211.25. In fact, training on GMPs is required for all new or temporary employees (eg, consultants, temps, project workers, etc.). GMP training is one training program that should be conducted annually for all employees (and others working

Table 4.4 Basic Quality Programs
Calibration
Change control
Cleaning
Document control
Preventive maintenance
Receiving
Sampling
Shipping
Training
Validation
Warehousing

on the site, eg, contractors) in order to remain current with all regulations. Training on SOPs is also required for new documents and whenever changes are made. The extent of the GMP training should be predicated on the job responsibilities. For example, anyone working in an aseptic area should have a full knowledge of the requirements for that area. This means more than just how to gown up appropriately.

All training programs should cover not only what needs to be done (or what shouldn't be done) but also provide the worker with some understanding of WHY it needs to be done and WHY done in that manner. This will help eliminate errors based on lack of understanding of the requirements.

Employees involved in the actual manufacturing of the product(s) need training in the operation of the equipment in their respective areas. They also need training on the SOPs directly and indirectly related to their job function (eg, filling out the batch record). The training program also needs to have a record of the training and the results of that training. These training records should be retained either by the Training Department or Human Resources.

BASIC RISK APPROACH[4]

A risk-based program needs to be established at the very beginning of the process validation program. Some criteria to be included in this risk program are:

- Documentation
- Security
- Training
- Equipment
- Process
- Changes (expected and other)

Starting a risk-based approach early in the development of the process, design, and implementation of the process is important to understand the risks involved in the process and to control the risks so as to limit unacceptable product production. Risk (to the product or patient) is often established through the use of the Failure Mode Effects Analysis, discussed further in Chapter 7, "Process Development." Rankings should be expressed as High, Medium, and Low. Items in the "high" category need to be addressed immediately and if not correctable monitored carefully. Those items in the "low" category can be addressed as needed, not ignored, but not considered a priority. Those in the "medium" category are in the middle and decisions have to be made on the priority status of them.

PUTTING IT TOGETHER

The discussion above has been about the documents needed for the completion of a process validation project. The general flow of a project is seen in Fig. 4.4. Now we turn to the actual setup of the project. First of all there has to be a lead (project manager) person. This person is responsible for assuring that all phases of the project are completed on time and on budget. They are also a team player, not just giving orders but helping resolve issues to move the project along. Other departments, not listed in this organization chart above, may also get involved at different times throughout the project (eg, Regulatory).

A scheduler will set the time line into a document, as seen in Fig. 4.5 (Gantt chart), that shows all the parts of the project and how they are related to each other in time. Purchasing will contract the vendors

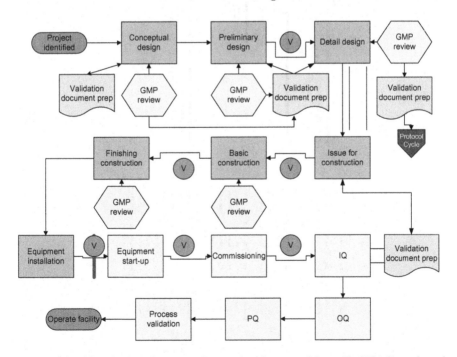

Figure 4.4 General flow plan for a pharmaceutical process through process validation. The "V" indicates the need for QA and/or QC involvement. Source: Informa Healthcare.

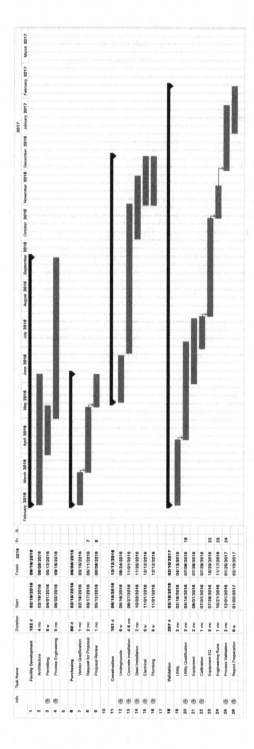

Figure 4.5 Gantt chart showing a sample project time line

(upon completing a vendor qualification program), with the requirements established by the process engineers, for the equipment, raw materials, etc. When the equipment arrives it needs to be installed (site acceptance test (SAT) may be performed, see Chapter 5, "Basic Equipment and Utility Qualification" and calibrated (Metrology Department), operators will need to be trained on the use of the equipment and the relevant SOPs,[5] and the Quality unit will work on documentation of the installation, facility development, etc.

Thus, it is clear that a process validation project can, and often does, take on many facets and involve many departments. Organization is critical to getting started, selecting the correct team leaders, training the staff, reviewing all documents, and establishing a risk-based, good science approach will result in a successful project.

In summary, to get started[6] efficiently the following is needed:

- Project Leader
  - Designated Team (eg, Fig. 4.1)
- Calibration
  - Process Equipment Instruments
  - Test Instruments (calibration needs to be before and after each test)
- User Specifications/Requirements
- Risk Analysis Completed[4]
  - Equipment
  - Process Steps (Criticality Determined)
- Utilities Commissioned/Qualified (as necessary depending on product contact and risk base to product)
- Process Equipment Qualified
- SOPs Written and Approved
- Protocol(s) Written and Approved
- Quality Systems In Place
- Personnel Trained
  - SOP
  - Equipment Operation
  - Recording Data—Protocol Execution
- Sufficient materials
  - Excipients
  - Active pharmaceutical ingredient
- Cleaning Verification (some do Cleaning Validation before)

NOTES

1. Pharmaceutical CGMPs for the 21st Century—A Risk-Based Approach Final Report; FDA, Sep. 2004.

2. Guidance for Industry; Q 10 Pharmaceutical Quality Systems Q10, FDA, Apr. 2009 ICH.

3. Guide to the Inspection of Quality Systems, FDA, Aug. 1999.

4. Guidance for Industry: Q9 Quality Risk Management, FDA, Jun. 2006 ICH.

5. Title 21 CFR 211.25, FDA, 2015.

6. Katz, P., Campbell, C.: FDA 2011 Process Validation Guidance: Process Validation Revisited. J. of GxP Compliance 16(4):18–29, 2012.

CHAPTER 5

Basic Equipment and Utility Qualification[1]

INTRODUCTION

Subpart D[2] of the Code of Federal Regulations is dedicated to equipment. 21 CFR 211.63 deals with design issues, 211.65 with construction, 211.67 and 68 deal with maintenance, cleaning, and automation. The one remaining section 211.72, deals with filters, types (no fibers), and uses. All of these are critical to assuring that the production of the product(s) remains in control and that they are consistent in identity, strength, quality, and purity.

Some consider equipment and utility qualification to be part of Stage II,[3] however, for our purpose it is included in Stage I. In reality, it does not matter in which stage it is included as long as it is completed prior to the execution of the process validation. The process cannot be validated unless all of the support utilities and the process equipment have first been qualified.

If the Active Pharmaceutical Ingredient (API) is known, then the manufacturer obtains it from a qualified vendor. If the API is not known and needs to be developed, the R&D department screens compounds and selects the most likely candidate (see Chapter 4: Getting Started). Once the moiety has been selected as a promising drug candidate the formulation team and process engineers begin their planning. The formulation department plans the means of the drug delivery (eg, tablet, parenteral, cream), the engineers take the information on the chemical and physical nature of the product and determine the equipment type to be used. That is, they are told the process needs (eg, blending, granulation, mixing, etc.). Marketing and the process group then determine the batch size needed. With this information the process engineers then work out the specifications for the equipment. This information is known as the user specifications or user requirements. The user specifications are then submitted to the vendors and bids are obtained.

How to Validate a Pharmaceutical Process. DOI: http://dx.doi.org/10.1016/B978-0-12-804148-2.00005-6

DETERMINING THE LEVEL OF QUALIFICATION

Before determining what testing needs to be performed in the Factory Acceptance Test (FAT) or any other commissioning or qualification test, one needs to determine the level of testing required. This is primarily determined by the amount of product contact and its criticality to the process. In determining the type and extent of the qualification needed for a particular piece of equipment the extent of its product contact needs to be considered:

- Direct Contact—comes in direct contact with the product or any of its components (eg, tanks)
- Indirect Contact—May come into product contact (eg, breathing air, a leak in an air-actuated valve)
- No Contact—There is no interaction by the equipment (eg, HVAC cooling tower)

Another consideration in determining the extent of testing required is "How critical is the equipment or its operation to the product?" Here criticality is defined as being necessary for the product to be produced correctly and consistently. For example, a tank is not a critical piece of equipment other than acting as a container for the product, yet a tank and agitator and controller for controlling the mixing time and speed can be critical in combination. The more critical the unit is to the process the more testing that needs to be performed. This is the beginning of the risk-based approach currently used by the FDA and other regulatory agencies.[4]

Qualification protocols need to test those parameters considered critical or necessary to the equipment's operation and/or function. Some equipment may have additional features that are not needed by the current process. Thus, if a unit has 10 functions but only 5 will ever be used, then only those 5 need to be qualified. However, all of the other unused functions must show that they do not interfere or compromise the functions that are to be used and that they are also "locked" out from any use. It is extremely important to note that until the unused functions are qualified, those functions cannot be used.

FACTORY ACCEPTANCE TEST AND SITE ACCEPTANCE TEST

As mentioned above, the user specifications are usually general in nature. For example, they would say we need a V blender with temperature control. The engineers would take this information and prepare the functional specifications. These would include the material of construction (usually stainless steel), how it was to be turned (ie, wall mounted or on the floor), and all the other technical specifications needed for the production or purchase of the unit. The functional specifications would be transmitted to the equipment manufacturer who would determine the design specifications, that is, how it was to be built to meet the user and functional specifications.

Once the equipment is built at the vendors shop the testing begins. FAT should be completed on all major equipment before they leave the vendors' facility. For example, large items (eg, autoclaves) will have a FAT performed. The purpose of the FAT test is for the vendor to demonstrate that the unit will meet the functions and design requirements specified when the order was placed. Be sure to have the vendor include testing that is applicable to your product, not just the tests that the equipment manufacture knows will pass. Very often the vendor will prepare the FAT protocol. However, it is strongly recommended that the drug manufacturer prepare at least some of the testing so as to be assured that the equipment meets their requirement, not just the vendors. These tests should also include the automation or control systems and software. Examples of some of the tests for a V blender are:

- Temperature and/or speed ramp up/down
- Hold or dwell times
- Speed/temperature control
- Stability or lack of vibration during maximum run conditions
- Pressure hold or leak tests
- Function of interlocks and other safety items.

Assuming the unit passes the FAT the unit is sent to the drug manufacturers site for installation.

Upon delivery to the manufacturing site the equipment vendor usually performs the installation of the equipment. After installation is complete a site acceptance test (SAT) would then be conducted (NOTE: Calibration of the units instruments should probably be completed at this stage to assure correct operation of the unit). This test is often very similar to the FAT (Note: Again, be sure specific tests related to your product are included) performed at the vendor's factory but may have additional tests included at the request of the drug manufacturer. It is used to confirm that the unit was not damaged, or pieces lost or loosened during shipment to the drug manufacturer's site.

Keep in mind that if documented correctly, and signed by trained observers, and with QA agreement some of the data collected in the FAT and/or SAT may be used to support the Installation Qualification (IQ) or Operational Qualification (OQ) protocols. Remember if this path is considered, the FAT and SAT documents need to be Good Manufacturing Practice (GMP) documents (Note: This is not a common practice). Successful completion of the FAT/SAT will save time in the end and gives the client the opportunity to make corrections to the specification or correct any miscommunication, or misinterpretation, of the user requirements.

The SAT should be completed before the vendor leaves the site and the final payment is made. The SAT may also include additional testing not performed at the vendor's factory. This test should not be confused with the IQ or OQ testing, which will be performed later. The focus of the prequalification testing is to make the vendor demonstrate that all components work properly. This may also be included in the commissioning activities discussed below.

COMMISSIONING

According to 21 CFR 211.63 the equipment and utilities need to be designed and located so as to allow the process to continue efficiently. During the commissioning phase of the equipment installation and start up, changes can be made to make the equipment more compatible to the process or to eliminate any defects not detected during installation. Commissioning usually follows the SAT; however, it may be combined with the SAT. Once the equipment has been installed and the SAT is complete (if performed) the vendor or manufacturer's staff can begin the commissioning of the unit. Commissioning is the step used to get the unit ready for use and to set or reset it for its function in the new pharmaceutical process. It is a written set of procedures used to prepare the equipment for qualification. For example, the control points, valves, and other functional components can be adjusted or "fixed" according to user or functional specifications in order to make the unit function more effectively. All changes made during commissioning need to be recorded. However, the commissioning document is not usually considered a Current Good Manufacturing Practice (CGMP) document (ie, approved by QU).

All components of the system that influence its functionality for the process are to be tested to ensure that the equipment will meet its expected operating criteria. Electrical or mechanical adjustments may be made in order to reach design-operating condition (eg, air pressures may be adjusted, valves replaced, or wiring fixed), and again these adjustments or changes must be recorded to provide an accurate record of the starting set points or operating conditions. The adjustments are made so that when the unit is qualified it will meet all requirements. This is why commissioning is considered a start-up operation and not a CGMP-regulated function.

Some commissioning activities are:

- "Bumping" the motors—checks for direction of rotation and speed. This verifies correct installation of the electrical components and polarity of the circuit.
- Adjusting flow rates—for example, in Water for Injection systems there is often an ozone generator for sanitization. The ozone flow needs to be adjusted so as to sanitize the systems and also have all the ozone removed prior to use in the drug manufacturing.
- Pressure testing the plumbing to demonstrate that the piping has been installed correctly and is leak free

It is advisable to include the Quality units input since many of the commissioning tests can be used for completing the IQ and OQ protocols. Fig. 5.1 shows a simple schematic to the qualification of equipment and utilities.

Utilities that have no direct product contact are usually only commissioned, not qualified. This also depends on the contact the system has with the product. Some examples of utilities that often have no direct impact on the product include the HVAC system (some exceptions, eg, aseptic/sterile area operations), electrical power, boiler steam, and cooling tower water.

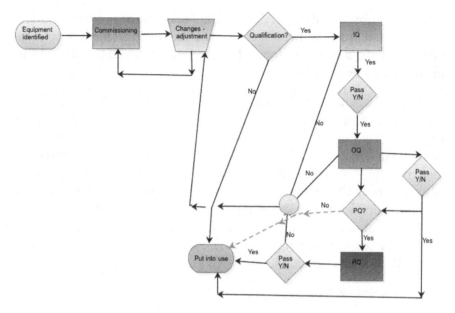

Figure 5.1 Equipment and utility qualification flow chart.

QUALIFICATION PROTOCOLS—INSTALLATION QUALIFICATION (IQ) AND OPERATIONAL QUALIFICATION (OQ)

The IQ and OQ documents are prepared as a protocol (test plan). These are CGMP documents and must be approved by the QU. These protocols must also be preapproved by relevant groups (eg, Operations, Engineering, Validation, Quality) prior to their execution and again (by the same functional groups or persons) upon completion of all testing. The purpose of the preapproval signatures is to have the protocols reviewed by the appropriate (involved) groups before execution and to indicate that they are in agreement with the tests to be performed. The signature following execution is to indicate that they approve of all the results and that the data are correct and acceptable. Each person reviewing and signing the preapproval should be reviewing the document from the perspective of their own specialty, that is, engineering reviews it for compliance to the engineering aspects, operations/manufacturing reviews it for its impact on the operators and the process (are all the buttons, controls, etc. there and accounted for), and QU reviews it for adherence to company and regulatory requirements. The protocol is closed by signing indicating that they are in agreement with the test results, and all deviations are closed. Only when all of the protocol components are complete will the approvers review the document and attest that all data are correct to the best of their understanding (ie, it appears correct, all completed, and any corrections are appropriate) and that the protocol is considered complete and ready for the final report.

Even following a complete, well documented, commissioning program the equipment still needs to be qualified. This has been done through the IQ and OQ. Today these are often joined into one document referred to as the Equipment Qualification (EQ). While the title does not matter, the content does. The equipment must be shown to meet the necessary requirements of the process. During the IQ/OQ or EQ testing each piece of equipment is operated independently (ie, tested so as to work as a stand alone system[5]) so as to demonstrate it can function as required. These tests are performed not only to show that the equipment meets the specifications required for the product but also those established by the equipment vendor so as to prolong the usefulness of the equipment. The IQ covers the physical attributes of the equipment or system. The OQ covers the operational aspects of the equipment or system. Tables 5.1 and 5.2 give some of the items to be tested or further documented in these documents.

One function of these protocols is to document the original installation conditions; and a second important function is to demonstrate that the equipment is suitable for the task to which it is assigned. The protocols need to be organized, easy to follow, and must "test" each major component or operation as it would impact the process. The IQ and OQ protocols are often referred to as "water runs." This is because the product need not be used in any of the tests (there are some exceptions, eg, high viscosity available only in the product).

Table 5.1 IQ—Physical Parameters of the System
• All required or identifiable major components are present
• Materials of construction—product contact areas only
• Make & model
• Capacity drawings and documents (to be made "as built")
• Weld and pressure test reports
• Spare parts list (parts needed to keep the equipment operational that would otherwise disable the machine for a long period of time)
• Lubricants/consumables list (use food grade lubricants)
• Utilities
• Connections
• Qualified/commissioned
• Room environment

Table 5.2 OQ—Operating Parameters/Function Tests

- System output versus design
  - Product flow
  - Speed control—in operation
  - Direction of operation (can be part of commissioning)
  - Calibration of system instruments
- Calibration of Test Instruments
- Controls, alarms and interlocks operation
- Utilities connections & pressure/flows
- System SOPs available (drafts are acceptable)
- System recovery after power failure
- Part 11 compliance
- System challenges
  - Cleaning
  - Full operation range
- Emergency power operation
- System suitability test
  - Functions for intended purpose
  - Functions as designed (user/functional specifications)
- Control functions
  - Ranges
    - Ramp up/down
      - Temperatures
      - Speed
      - Pressure

The above IQ and OQ tests can be lumped together into usable categories necessary to demonstrate effectiveness of both construction and operations such as:

- Materials of construction—the materials, according to 21 CFR 211.65, "... shall not be reactive, additive, or absorptive so as to alter the safety, strength, quality, or purity of the drug product ..." In addition it goes on to refer to the lubricants or coolants used should not interfere with the drug product. Thus, the use of food grade lubricants is considered standard practice.
- System Suitability—21 CFR Subpart D deals with this aspect of the equipment. This covers both the physical and operational characteristics of the equipment. The equipment should function for its intended purpose and be of the correct size (eg, usually 50–75% greater capacity than required so as to prevent overflows, or its reduce duty cycle).
- Operating Ranges—the equipment should be tested for operation over its full range. This accomplishes two things, one is the equipment is shown to be able to run at all speeds or conditions, and two, prevents the need to retest or further demonstrate that the

equipment will operate at other speeds or conditions at a later time when additional products are added to the system.

- Installation Reports—these would include items such as the weld reports, materials of construction, surface finish, pressure or leak testing of piping or ductwork. Also included would be verification of the level of the equipment, the distance from the wall or floor as specified by the manufacturer.

Performance Qualification[6]

The Performance Qualification (PQ) are those tests that are performed as a process train or operations and are performed on critical units or systems that usually function as a group and not individually. However, some single units may also require PQ tests depending on their impact on the product. Examples of these are water systems (utilities), packaging lines (production), or autoclaves/steam sterilizers (production). The PQ protocol usually requires the product to be used for the testing. This is to demonstrate that the units, together, can perform as expected and produce the product. Now that each major component has been qualified in the IQ and OQ stage, the complete system must be run as expected. The format for a PQ protocol is similar to an OQ protocol and is as follows (Table 5.3):

LABORATORY EQUIPMENT QUALIFICATION (EQ)

Laboratory equipment used in the release or testing of pharmaceutical products (or intermediates), with the exception of basic research laboratory equipment, must be qualified prior to its use (just as one would qualify the process equipment). Since this equipment is used to determine the status or release of the product (or intermediates) either to the next process step or for release for commercial distribution, it needs to be fully qualified and calibrated so that there is no question as to the results obtained. If the calibration, preventive maintenance, or qualification is

Table 5.3 Table of Contents of a PQ Protocol

- Approvals
- Purpose
- Responsibilities
- References
- Process description
- Test for process parameters
- Acceptance criteria
- Results

incomplete or not performed prior to use the test results could be called into question. Although most laboratory instruments (equipment) often stand alone, there are some instruments that are "on-line." These instruments also must be qualified prior to use and can be included with the process unit with which they are associated. The product passes through these on-line instruments and the results are available immediately (eg, Process Analytical Technology[7]—PAT operations).

Often the equipment vendor supplies the qualification protocols for laboratory equipment. These documents are a good starting point but often need to be supplemented with additional tests or conditions specific for the expected laboratory or process use. The qualification program for laboratory equipment is the same as for process equipment. An IQ and an OQ are needed. PQs are not as common, but certainly are performed for some equipment (eg, autoclave and glassware washers).

QUALIFICATION PROTOCOL EXECUTION

When all of the equipment is ready (commissioned, calibrated, and available) and the protocols approved, the protocols can then be executed. For this the staff needs to be trained on how to execute the protocol (a Standard operating procedure—SOP) and how to operate the equipment. It also may be necessary to have other specialists available to perform specialty tests (eg, electrician or plumber).

The IQ and OQ can be executed simultaneously, however, the IQ must be completed (approved) prior to the approval of the OQ. Table 5.4 shows some of the things that should be in place prior to executing a qualification protocol.

The execution of the PQ protocols is again similar to that of the IQ or OQ. Trained operators are needed to run the equipment, and sufficient test material is needed for the testing. It is best to run the tests

---

Table 5.4 Basic Check List Before IQ/OQ/PQ Execution

- All test instruments are calibrated and must remain in calibration during all testing
- Process equipment instrumentation has been calibrated
- Protocols are preapproved prior to execution
  - System boundaries are complete
- Personnel are trained on the equipment operation and the protocol tests
- Sufficient test material is available
- Piping and instrument drawings (P&ID) are issued for construction and become "as built" following execution (if not before)

starting with the lowest concentration or speed and build up to maximum operation. This allows for conservation of materials. Also, it may minimize cleaning or set-up times between runs. The appropriate individuals (ie, those who preapproved the protocols) must carefully review all data and a final report prepared. This report can be incorporated into the IQ and OQ report or may stand alone to represent the final acceptance of the unit(s). From the CFR it is clear that the equipment and utilities need to be ready for use prior to performing the process validation.

Reports

Summary reports must be prepared upon completion of the execution of the protocols. The reports may be combined for the IQ and OQ, or they may be independent documents (ie, stand-alone). A final report closes out the protocol regardless of pass or fail. If the unit fails, the team needs to determine why (see Chapter 9: Dealing With Deviations). As stated they may be attached to the protocols, or prepared as stand-alone documents, to be presented to the regulatory agencies without the encumbrance of the supporting data. Of course, either way, all supporting data and tests must be available upon request. The same people who approved the protocol must also approve the report.

Calibration and Preventive Maintenance Programs[8]

As mentioned earlier in this chapter, before a process unit can be put into use it has to have calibrated instruments. This needs to be part of a program that traces all calibrations to be performed. With this program the date of all calibrations is tracked and any miss is considered a deviation and must be investigated. There are many software programs available for this purpose. The calibration program includes all test instruments and all instrumentation on or functioning with the process equipment or utility. It is taken as industry standard that critical process instruments are to be calibrated at least twice a year (every 6 months). However, there is no official regulation for this. Calibration should be checked to assure that the instrument remains in calibration for the time required (1 day or 1 year). Noncritical instruments can have longer calibration times but this needs to be verified. As an example, a temperature gauge on an autoclave would start with a calibration at first use, then at 1 month, and every month thereafter. Assuming it remains in calibration for a period of 4 months the calibration can then be checked at 3-month intervals. This would hold for all instruments, critical or noncritical. In any case, critical instruments need to be calibrated on a regular basis (usually 3–6 months).

The preventive maintenance program is similar to the calibration program. It is usually based on the equipment manufacturers recommendations. This program also needs to be qualified or validated. As above, start with short-term testing of the maintenance and extend it as the equipment allows (if there is no equipment vendor recommendation).

The FDA considers both of these programs core quality programs. Full documentation and investigations for missed dates are required.

NOTES

1. Ostrove, S.: Qualification and Change Control. In: Validation of Pharmaceutical Processes, 3rd Ed; Editors: Agalloco, J., Carlton, F. New York: Informa Healthcare USA, Inc., 2008, Chapter 9, pp. 129–145.

2. Title 21 CFR Part 211 Subpart D, FDA, 2015.

3. Process Validation A Life Cycle Approach; Grace McNally; FDA May 2011 slide presentation on www.FDA.gov

4. Guidance for Industry Process Validation: General Principles and Practices, FDA, Jan. 2011.

5. Stand alone system—several components working as a single unit of operation (eg, a pump and a tank).

6. Note: This is often combined with part of the process performance qualification and may become a part of the validation teams' efforts (whereas the IQ and OQ testing are often performed by the engineering group).

7. Guidance for Industry: PAT—A Framework for Innovative Pharmaceutical Development, Manufacturing and Quality Assurance, FDA, Sep. 2004.

8. Bringert, G.: Calibration and Metrology, In: Validation of Pharmaceutical Processes, 3rd Ed; Editors: Agalloco, J., Carlton, F. New York: Informa Healthcare USA, Inc., 2008, Chapter 7, pp. 99–108.

CHAPTER 6

Computers and Automated Systems

INTRODUCTION

This chapter will provide an overview of how computer controlled or automated units are to be qualified and then validated as part of and included with process systems. Note that while each is discussed as operational units standing alone, they can and should be qualified and/or validated as part of the process equipment they are associated with when those units are qualified. This chapter is not intended to be a full tutorial on computer validation. The use of the terms "qualified" and "validated" are used and applied, as they normally would be (ie, equipment—hardware is qualified; and the process—software working with the hardware is validated). Remember, when qualifying a computer controlled system you are also "validating" both the computer system and the process equipment. Both the structure and function of the computer and the process equipment are all to be done at the same time.

The US Food and Drug Administration (FDA) considers computer systems as equipment 21 CFR 211.68[1] and thus needs to be formally qualified. The use of computerized control for manufacturing and quality control has grown substantially over the last few decades. The FDA has published guidelines on computer software validation (including Part 11).[2] In addition, the GAMP[3] (Good Automated Manufacturing Practice) guideline has been adopted as the standard for most computer systems validation (CSV) programs. There are five (really now only 4) levels of systems according to the GAMP 5[4] guide, these are:

- Category 1—Infrastructure Software—Operating systems, database managers, statistical programing tools, and programming languages.
- Category 2—NO LONGER IN USE BY GAMP 5.
- Category 3—Nonconfigurable Product—Nonconfigurable, also called "Off the Shelf" used for business purposes.

How to Validate a Pharmaceutical Process. DOI: http://dx.doi.org/10.1016/B978-0-12-804148-2.00006-8

- Category 4—Configurable Product—Standardized packages that the owner can configure to fit their specific needs or operations. These can perform a general function, for example, blending. These are termed COTS or "Configurable Off The Shelf."
- Category 5—Custom Application—Prepared specifically for the operation (usually prepared by specialty firms or in-house programmers).

Each level above requires its own level of qualification. Using a current risk-based approach to the qualification, as the level increases more testing is necessary. Notice that the levels are primarily related to the software and not the hardware. This is because the hardware serves only as the framework in which the software performs its function. The interaction and function of the software and hardware must also be qualified; that is, it is not possible to qualify one without the other.

This area has become more important over the last several years since all, or certainly most, pieces of equipment used in the manufacture of pharmaceutical products have some form of computer control. These range from microchips to full computer systems with interactive screen control for the operator (eg, SCADA).

Yet another aspect of computers and automated systems that is becoming a bigger part of process design is the use of Process Analytical Technology (PAT),[5] that is, automated feedback to more accurately control step(s) in the process.

Automated or computer controlled systems or their components and systems are often part of, or under the control of, the Process Automation or Information Technology (IT) department. They have the expertise in maintaining the systems and providing the necessary service and training to allow the end user (operations) to safely use the system effectively. This group certainly can and should be called on when validating a computer-controlled system (regardless of the level of computer control).

In addition, many (or most) computerized units can be linked into a network so that each is monitored by a higher level system that keeps each unit operational within its specifications and records the results of operations.

Table 6.1 Documents to Be Prepared or Made Available

1. CS-VMP—Computer system validation master plan
2. User requirements/specifications
3. Number of system users
4. Functional specifications
5. Traceability matrix—(Note: To be prepared AFTER all specifications and protocols have been collected and developed but BEFORE protocol execution)
6. General SOPs needed
   a. System setup/installation
   b. Data collection and handling
   c. System maintenance
   d. Data backup (data integrity testing)
   e. Recovery
      i. Crash
      ii. Freeze
   f. Emergencies
   g. Security (especially if Part 11 is used)
   h. Change control
   i. Data storage/recovery (current and backup data)
7. Protocols
   a. Commissioning
   b. IQ
   c. OQ
   d. PQ (as necessary)

Collect (as possible):
1. Source code
   a. Ladder logic (for PLCs)
2. Design or Vendor specifications for each component—part of the system (network interfacing, man—machine interfacing; MMI)
3. Software version to be installed

GENERAL CONSIDERATIONS[6]

Documentation

When beginning a CSV program, as with other qualification programs, certain documents need to be either prepared or collected. Since the qualification will involve components not usually seen, and/or not usually accessible, having the correct documents at the very beginning of the project will help assure its success. Table 6.1 lists some of the main documents to be prepared or collected:

Testing

In general, software qualification, as discussed below, requires vigorous testing along with its associated hardware. This testing needs to include the actual operation of the field instruments (valves, etc.), as well as the recording and storage of the data generated.[7] Any changes in the contents of the systems (including the wires that connect the field instruments to the computer) need to be included in the change control program (see chapter: The Validation Life Cycle and Change Control).

Software qualification is usually separated into two distinct activities; the structural testing and the functional testing. The structural testing includes the vendor audit, review of the code, and checks on the integrity of the code, for example, so that there is no dead code (ie, nonoperational code that may cause a "crash" or data error). The functional testing is just as the name implies, testing the functionality of the operation of each part or software function.

Basic CSV[8]—Black Box—Gray Box—White Box Testing

There are three methods of testing computer control or automated systems. These are referred to as "White box," "Gray Box," and "Black Box" testing. The difference between "white" and "black" box testing is in the level of functional testing of the software. Black box testing is primarily functional testing only. When carrying out black box testing the operation of each portion of the software is tested. White box testing includes complete structural testing ie, review of the source code (of the software program) as well as the means of code development. In addition, the testing establishes that each function is necessary for the correct operation of the unit(s). Typically, the black box testing grows exponentially with the amount of I/O while the white box testing grows linearly.

A middle approach is "gray box" testing. As the name implies this is between the full white box and black box testing programs. Some structural tests will be performed yet the emphasis is on functional testing. Most equipment that contains a PLC or other controller is usually tested using gray box or black box testing while the higher-level control systems usually undergo more white box testing and more functional testing.

Computer Life Cycle

Computer controlled systems have basic similarities to other process components or systems. The life cycle approach is also applicable to computer systems, as seen below. GAMP 5 outlines these as:

- Concept—establishing system requirements
- Project—GxP (GMP, Part 11, etc.) assessment and release

- Operation—part of the full qualification program where a qualified state needs to be maintained
- Retirement—decommissioning the system for replacement by another system

Structural validation (analogous to the Installation Qualification (IQ) for equipment) occurs mainly in the concept and project stages while functional validation falls mostly into the project and operation, as well as the retirement stage.

Software qualification should start with a source code review, if possible (this is an IQ test).[9] This review includes vendor audits, review for dead code, annotation, etc. Keep in mind that it is not possible to do a line-by-line review of the code due to the number of lines of code. It may be possible (or necessary) to make arrangements with a third party, or the source code developer, to make code changes if it is found to be necessary during validation activities.

The second part of qualifying the code is its functional testing (analogous to the Operational Qualification (OQ)) for equipment. Thus, functional qualification of the software follows the same pattern as any other pharmaceutical equipment or systems qualification. In addition, as already mentioned, functional testing needs to include the interaction with the hardware of the computer system.

Today it is very common to include CSV functional and structural testing into the equipment EQ protocol rather than have it as a separate protocol. This enables the unit to be fully qualified both on its own and under the control system. In addition to the "usual" requirements for IQs and OQs the qualification of computer systems requires some additional items. Some of these are:

- Verification of System Security
  - Controlled access to the program
  - Levels of access—for example, an operator is allowed to input data but the supervisor is allowed to approve the data
  - Protection of the system from outside interference—(eg, no access via phone lines or the internet or ElectroMagnetic Interference (EMI), and/or Radio Frequency Interference (RFI)).

Note: Usually an intranet connection will be allowed through a secure firewall or intranet setup
- Data Integrity verification including storage and retrieval of the data
- Part 11 compliance—for example, and audit trail (eg, The ability to track all entries into the system—this includes the date, the person making the entry, and why the entry is made or changed)

As with all qualification programs the commissioning phase usually is the first "field" effort undertaken. (Note: This follows any FAT and SAT performed on the equipment). The commissioning portion of the qualification can be performed, at least in part, during the installation of the system. For example, while the lines are being run to the field instruments (if any) the loop checks can be performed. A loop check is a check of continuity (and thereby function) of the connection between a field instrument and the controller. It is far simpler to perform and document the loop check as each loop is being installed rather than after the system is intact and ready to operate. Other items that can be performed during the installation or as part of the commissioning phase are:

- Instruments Adjusted/Calibrated (Loop checks)
- Ambient Conditions
  - Temperature
  - Humidity
- Alarms and Events (general testing—operational testing is left to the OQ phase of the qualification)
- Graphics
- Database Location
- Network Configuration

The general the CSV IQ consists of the following verifications. Specific tests will be pointed out later for each of the types of auto-mated systems (Table 6.2).

In the case of automated systems, the completion of the IQ is necessary since the system will not function as specified without all components being installed correctly. While the system may seem to operate, some functions will be compromised if a component is lacking. This may not be immediately apparent but will, in the long term, compromise the final product. An example of this would be a missing printer. The controller would run, the

Table 6.2 IQ (Computer Physical Components and Software Structural Testing)

1. List all major components
   a. Input devices—Human Machine Interface (HMI)
      i. Keyboard
      ii. Mouse
      iii. External devices
         1. Field instruments,
         2. External drive or flash drives ports
         3. Monitors, etc.
   b. Output devices and data storage devices
      i. Screen
      ii. External data device—hard drive, flash drives, CD/DVD
      iii. Printer(s)
      iv. Filed instruments
   c. Mother board—chip type and /or serial number
   d. Controller and cards
      i. Video
      ii. Sound
      iii. I/O (input/output)
      iv. Serial
      v. S Video
      vi. Other monitor connections
      vii. Connection types (ports, etc.)
   e. Network configuration
2. Check for:
   a. Tight connections
   b. Correct component type
   c. Installed in the correct location (as applicable)
   d. Make and model as per specifications
3. Power (source and distribution)
   a. Volts
   b. Current
   c. Stability
   d. Surge protection
4. Software (includes the structural testing—see Note below)
   a. Version installed
   b. Source code verification
      i. Annotation
      ii. Dead code
      iii. Vendor testing verification (part of vendor audit)
   c. Compliance to good software preparation[2]

machines would run, but the output data would not be able to be expressed or recorded. This may cause the system to shut down or to store the information (usually in RAM—Random Access Memory—which is not permanent) that cannot be printed. It may be possible to be printed later. This may compromise the next lot of material being produced since it will get the incorrect label or printout. It is during the OQ testing that the software undergoes its functional testing (Table 6.3).

In preparing and testing the Performance Qualification (PQ) (Table 6.4) of the computer controls the following is usually included:

Table 6.3 OQ (Functional Testing of the Hardware and Software)
1. Prepare test of each component listed in the IQ
a. Meets design specifications
b. Meets functional specifications hardware
c. Power limits—may be included as part of the PQ (below)
i. Recovery after power loss
ii. Power line stability
d. Environmental stress
e. Alarms
f. All component functions over their full range
g. Software
i. Version verification
ii. Software serial number
iii. Ladder logic or source code review
h. Input limits (boundaries—number of operators allowed on at any given time)
i. Compete structural testing
j. Functional testing
i. Restart after shutdown
ii. Restart after power loss
iii. All major operations function and results are appropriate
2. RFI (Radio Frequency Interference)—that is a radio frequency should not cause the controller to malfunction (allow incorrect data in or out), for example, a walkie-talkie (hand held radios)
3. EMI (Electromagnetic Interference)—a magnetic field should not interfere with the data integrity, for example, an electric drill
4. I/O integrity
5. Calibration

Table 6.4 PQ (Performance Testing of the System(s))
1. Power failure recovery—computer & process equipment (as seen above this may be done as part of the OQ)
• Recovery after power loss
2. Security—system accessibility (Part 11 analysis and test)
• Password challenge
• Security challenge
• Biometric security
• Levels of access
3. Archive/retrieve data in real time
4. Produce batch report
5. Data lines transmission
6. General data integrity
7. Interference between programs/components
8. Software
• Full operation of all functions in conjunction with the entire system
• Stress the software boundaries
• Noninterference between modules or other programs

SPECIFIC SYSTEMS

The next part of this chapter will deal with some of the specific requirements needed to complete an adequate qualification of different types of automated systems. As was seen above, computer or automated control systems require both software and hardware qualification. The software qualification has adopted the GAMP approach while the hardware has retained the basic IQ/OQ/PQ approach. The specific types of systems that will be discussed are:

- Microprocessors
- Programmable Logic Controllers (PLCs)
- Personal Computers (PCs)
- Networks
- Supervisory Control and Data Acquisition—(SCADA)
- Distributed Control System (DCS)—all forms

Microprocessors

These controllers exist throughout the pharmaceutical industry. Their purpose is usually a single function such as turning the unit on or off, or controlling a light or a valve on a schedule. They are more than simple switches in that some have limited programing capabilities. Other examples of microprocessor controllers are:

- A door not closing within a set period of time may trigger an alarm
- Events (eg, labels attached, bottles sealed) may be counted

However, a microprocessor may be more advanced, that is, an Electronically Programmed Random Only Memory (EPROM) or it may be a little more sophisticated and is an electronically erasable (EEPROM). Both the EPROM and the EEPROM require software qualification as well as the standard functional testing of the microprocessor. The software to make these changes is accessible only through another computer and even then only with specialized software.

Microprocessor controlled equipment (eg, digital thermometer, barcode readers, pumps, interlock mechanisms, sensor activity) are usually validated only using black box testing, since the source code (program) is not available or accessible for any direct testing.

Programmable Logic Controllers (PLCs)

In the pharmaceutical industry, the PLC is probably the mainstay of all operations. The PLC can be found in a variety of operating units (eg, Autoclaves). They are used to open or close any type of field device (ie, valves, air pressure control, motors). In general, they are relatively easy to program (hence the name).

The PLC can be viewed as multiple microprocessors in a single unit. It typically has much more memory, and processing power than the microprocessor. Typically PLC code (called ladder logic as opposed to source code used for PCs and higher types of controllers) and hardware wiring are customized for each device based on the customer's specific needs. Because the code is to be customized by the client (operating company), the PLC manufacturers testing of the operating system software is usually only on a high level. This leaves the true qualification work to the owner.

From a risk assessment standpoint, PLCs typically have the highest direct safety risk (both human and equipment). For a simple PLC controller, for example, less than 20 input/outputs (I/O), black box testing makes more sense than white box. However, for anything more than 20 I/O or for systems with a Human Machine Interface (HMI), white box testing is probably more effective than black box testing. The amount and type of testing is related to the amount of code, the amount of user specified coding versus vendor coding, the actual use in the process (ie, what equipment it will be used to control), and other factors as outlined in the GAMP guide.

An example of PLC qualification can be seen as follows:

Assume that a machine has two sensors, A & B. When sensor A is on, we want to turn on alarm horn A. In addition, when sensor B is on, we want to turn on alarm horn B. However, if sensors A and B are on (horn A and B), we want to shut down the machine. The programmer can cause sensor A to set a bit that causes the output alarm horn A to turn on; and to set a bit so sensor B that causes the output alarm horn B to turn on. When both of these bits are on, the machine should stop.

Another example, assume we have a system of 5 inputs and 5 outputs. For the short term, we'll ignore the complexities that can be built into the operator interface. Given an input, or combination of inputs, some output(s) occur. Let's say that input 1, vessel pressure high, causes output 1 vessel vent valve, to actuate. The requirements and design documents will probably state, "Open the vessel vent valve when the vessel pressure is high." Most protocols would include a single test - stimulate the input, observe the response output. This must be done for each of the I/Os.

Table 6.5 Items to Verify for PLC's
• Review the ladder logic
◦ Correct version installed
• Inputs and outputs
• Environmental conditions
• Point to point testing—loop checks

Of course, as more interlocks, sequences, and other rules are added to the complexity of the PLC logic, the advantages are harder to see—though they are still there (Table 6.5).

Personal Computers

PCs such as laptops or desktop computers are more sophisticated than PLCs but are still relatively easy to qualify. The reason for this is that most of the software used on a PC is "off the shelf" nonconfigurable. That is, the software code cannot be changed. Only the application is configurable. For example, the Microsoft Excel spreadsheet program can neither be validated nor qualified. However, the application of each spreadsheet must be qualified. Specifically each calculation needs to be verified from both its algorithm to its data input and output.

All aspects of the PC need to be qualified, just as any other process or laboratory equipment. All input/output devices (eg, keyboards, disk drives, USB inputs of outputs, mouse control and other pointers, screen displays, printers, etc.) need to be tested and demonstrated to be functioning correctly. This means that the data being input is the same as the data coming out. For example, if you want to type the letter "M," the keyboard should only respond to the "M" key and the screen should display only an "M" from that designated key. The same holds true for data storage devices, whether internal or external.

Data storage devices also are part of the PC qualification program. Storage time of the data on the external device, as well as the environmental conditions it is stored under are factors in this qualification.

Operating systems are not usually qualified due to the large number of users. However, the vendor audit or other review for code preparation, annotation, etc. should be performed (Table 6.6).

Table 6.6 Items to Verify on a PC

- All input devices
- All output or data storage devices
- Data integrity both in and out of the PC
- PC calibration
- Software:
  - Operating and off the shelf programs do not usually require qualification
  - Application software and applications on off the shelf programs do require qualification (eg, COTS—Customizable Off The Shelf software)
- Environmental conditions—temperature/humidity/liquids

Table 6.7 Items to Consider for Network Qualification

- All major components of the network (eg, PCs, routers, switches)
  - Point to point testing
  - Quality of the signal
- Use the risk assessment approach to determine the extent of a network qualification
  - Transport layers
  - Application layers
- Commissions to specifications
- Validates to requirements
- Security (refer also to Part 11)
  - Open system
  - Closed systems
- Collision reconciliation
- Node operation

Networks

PLCs and PCs may be linked together to form a "Network." Simply, a network is a group of individual units (PCs or PLCs) linked together so that information can be easily shared. There are two basic types of networks—open and closed. In the pharmaceutical industry, the closed network is the preferred type.

If users transmit data over a network, then the network should be validated. However, that validation is usually a subset of validation of the database system (with tests that make sure clients can talk to servers and so forth). In addition, there is typically some platform validation performed to ensure that the network can handle traffic flow correctly.

A risk assessment should truly answer when and how to do network validation. For example, if the network is only used for backing up servers, then the firm would develop a set of requirements, specifications, and tests regarding how servers are backed up. If the network were only used for client interaction to the server, then the firm would develop requirements, specifications, and tests around network loading, response speed, and server timeouts (Table 6.7).

Supervisory Control and Data Acquisition (SCADA)

SCADA systems are made up of several components. Each of these components may be qualified as separate units or combined into one large qualification program. A SCADA system is made up of:

- HMI—The screen is often a touch screen
- Control Units—Controlling the field devices
- Main Processor—Interprets the information form the field units/PLCs and the operating instructions from the HMI

As with all automated or computerized systems, security and data integrity are primary issues. Each of the components needs to be secure from outside interference as well as internal problems resulting from adjacent equipment or component problems. Alarms are also key to the functioning of a SCADA system. They alert the operator to problems in carrying out the instructions made by the operator or the recipe (Table 6.8).

Distributed Control Systems (DCS)

Distributed control systems (DCS) have evolved over the years. These systems are involved in more than just pharmaceutical manufacturing. They are found in inventory control, warehousing, ordering, maintenance, and manufacturing controls. Building Management Systems (BMS), Materials Resource Planning Systems (MRP), and Enterprise

---

Table 6.8 Items to Verify for a SCADA Qualification

- Alarms
- Loop checks
  - Point to point are unique
  - Field unit verifications
- Input devices
  - Human Machine Interface
    - Access levels
      - Supervisor
      - Operator
  - Disks
  - Tapes
- Graphics
  - Is the system represented correctly on the screen
- Data acquisition and data integrity
- Is the screen a true representation of the system
- Is it a touch screen?
- Interface between the screen and the system (ie, valves, temperature control, etc.).
  - Does the screen do what is indicated in the system
- Calibration

Table 6.9 Items to Verify for a DCS

• Individual node/unit can function independently
  • No interference between units
  • No interference between users
• Each node/unit can be qualified independently
• Environmental conditions for each node
• Input and out devices
• Network qualification
• HMI qualification

Resource Planning (ERP) are examples of DCS systems. These systems integrate many functions into one package. The BMS controls and monitors the environmental conditions in the facility. It can prepare documentation on the environmental status of any part of the plant if requested or as part of a batch record. It can monitor the fire alarms or access to restricted areas. MRP and ERP systems are used for complete inventory and manufacturing control (Table 6.9).

PART 11

No discussion of computer or control system qualification will be complete without at least an overview of Part 11 (21 CFR Part 11[10]). This part of the CFR has caused the pharmaceutical industry great concern in recent years due to its perceived complexity. Part 11 has been around since 1997 and is being implemented more effectively due to the revised guidelines.[11] According to the latest guidelines, systems put into operation prior to Aug. 1997 are considered exempt from the Part 11 rules. However, caution needs to be taken here, as any change to the system after the 1997 start, may bring the control system under Part 11 requirements.

The emphasis of Part 11 is to assure that only authorized personnel enter data, review the data, and/or change the data. All changes to the data needs to have an explanation, just as error corrections on paper require a note explaining the reason for the change. This notation is referred to as the audit trail. Care must be taken in the selection of software that includes a secure audit trail if electronic records are to be used.

Subparts B and C (of 21 CFR Part 11) represent the main body of the requirements. Only an overview of the requirements will be presented here; further study will be required to fully understand this section of the CFR.

Subpart B is concerned with any computerized system. Both open and closed systems are included (11 CFR 11.10 and 11 CFR 11.30). In this part of the CFR the FDA specifies that any system used to "create, modify, maintain, or transmit electronic records shall employ procedures and controls designed to ensure the authenticity, integrity ... and ensure that the signer cannot readily repudiate the signed record as not genuine."[12] This means that the system(s) need to be validated/ qualified and that, as with written records, there needs to be traceability of all data. Access to the systems and the data or records (electronic) needs to be limited to authorized personnel only.

Records that are maintained in paper format, as the final official copy, are not included in this section of the regulations. Paper records are part of what is known as the predicate rules requirements. The predicate rules are any rule previously established as found in 21 CFR Part 211.

Subpart C deals with the actual control and requirements for electronic signatures. It describes the levels for security and access, the need for verification of the person signing. There are two types of identification discussed; these are, biometric and nonbiometric. The nonbiometric form is most familiar to everyone. These include items such as user identification, identification badges (picture ID) sign-in logs, and passwords. If this type of identification is used, then two forms must accompany the signature (ie, user identification and a password). On the other hand, a biometric identification requires only one means of identification and verification of the user. These include fingerprint identity, retinal scans of the eye, or voice recognition. Biometric identification is becoming easier and less expensive, and is available on some PCs now.

As can be seen from this short discussion of Part 11, the regulations are not difficult, however, some aspects of the rules may be harder to implement. All control systems have, or should have, limited access to both the system and the various levels of data (eg, operator, supervisor, and administrator). Any change in the data needs to have a "trail" indicating "who" made the change and why the change was made (similar to changes in paper records). Thus, compliance to Part 11 has become achievable and, with the new Guidelines from the FDA, it has become more understandable. However, care needs to be taken with all computerized systems to be sure that all of the Part 11 regulations are implemented.

NOTES

1. Title 21 CFR 211.68.

2. General Principles of Software Validation; Final guidance for Industry and FDA Staff, FDA, Jan. 2002. Guidance for Industry Part 11 Electronic Records; Electronic Signatures – Scope and Application, FDA, Feb. 2003.

3. GAMP Guide for Validation of Automated Systems, Ed. 4, ISPE 2001.

4. GAMP 5 A Risk-Based Approach to Compliant GxP Computerized Systems, ISPE, 2008.

5. Guidance for Industry: PAT—A Framework for Innovative Pharmaceutical Development, Manufacturing and Quality Assurance, FDA, Sep. 2004.

6. Ostrove, S.: Qualification and Change Control. In: Validation of Pharmaceutical Processes, 3rd Ed; Editors: Agalloco, J, Carlton, F. New York: Informa Healthcare USA, Inc., 2008, Chapter 46, pp. 619–628-145.

7. Data Integrity and Compliance with CGMP, Guidance for Industry, FDA, April, 2016.

8. Technical Report No. 18; Validation of Computer Related Systems, Parenteral Drug Association, 49(S1); 1995.

9. NOTE: Ladder logic and source codes need to be reviewed for compliance to good code writing requirements. Two of the items that should be included in this review are a review for dead code (ie, code that has no use but may cause errors in the program when run) and annotation. Ladder logic (the programming code used for PLCs) should be reviewed for functionality as well as annotations. While the source code of higher systems (PCs, etc.) also needs to be reviewed (eg, for dead code but also for annotation of the sections).

10. Title 21 CFR Part 11, 2015.

11. Part 11 guidelines.

12. Title 21 CFR 11.10, 201.

STAGE II—PROCESS DEVELOPMENT

CHAPTER 7

Process Development*

PRELIMINARIES

Before a process validation program can begin one has to clearly define the process. This means that all of the process equipment needs to be defined as to size and expected function. It also means that the chemistry of the process needs to have a clear definition. Intermediates, reaction rates, control points, end points to reactions, etc. need to be considered and included in the developmental workup of the process. In Chapter 4, "Getting Started," the role of the research and the development departments were briefly discussed. In this chapter we will delve more deeply into their function as well as the function of the Development department/group.

The medicinal chemistry[1] group designs a compound (moiety) that will either inhibit or stimulate a biochemical process in the body. The research department's (usually R&D) function is to screen these compounds either in vitro or in vivo (in a living organism) to determine which, if any, of the moiety's supplied by the medicinal chemistry group have biological activity worth further testing.

Once the research group has determined that a molecule (moiety) is found to be active in producing the results needed for pharmacological action (it can be either a positive or negative affect) it is passed to the development group. It may also be sent to the isolation/purification department. In both of these areas the moiety is further developed and "cleaned." The reason for this is to obtain one molecule that has the necessary properties for its intended pharmacological action. While the purification work is going on, the development group is studying its properties for possible commercial production. The research group is also continuing its studies on the compound (eg, biochemical action or specificity, toxicity, etc.). The work that is going on at this phase is to determine the chemical properties that will enable production at a large scale.

*Bold text in this chapter is by the author for clarity only.

How to Validate a Pharmaceutical Process. DOI: http://dx.doi.org/10.1016/B978-0-12-804148-2.00007-X

For example, prior to the advent of the statin drugs, that reduce the production of cholesterol, research groups screened hundreds of moieties in vitro (e.g., cell culture) for anti-cholesterol biosynthesis activity. Those compounds that showed activity in reducing the amount of cholesterol produced were sent for further testing. That is, looking for its mode of action and further defining the range of inhibition that could be expected. Activity curves, specific activity, action in other parts of the sterol pathway, impact on other aspects of the cell biochemistry were also studied.[2]

In most cases the first part of development is to determine the range of activity of the moiety. That is, what is the highest and lowest concentration that will yield an effective response? While this titration work is going on, the development group is working on scaling up the work. Compounds that are tested in basic research are usually produced in very small quantities (ie, laboratory scale). Thus, in order to do additional testing (eventually clinical trials) larger quantities need to be produced. This is the job of the development group. Fig. 7.1 shows a schematic flow of the process to get to the Process Performance Qualification (PPQ).

DEVELOPMENT

Some of the information the medicinal chemistry departments should be able to supply to the R&D group as they start development workup is:

- Source of the moiety
- Name, structure, and class of the active moiety
- Physical properties—for example, solubility in water, solvents, etc.
  - pK_a, pH, etc.
  - Stability
    - Temperature—boiling point, freezing point, etc.
    - Duration—how long it is stable under specified conditions,
    - Best/Worst conditions—for example, stable when concentrated or dilute
- Chemical properties
  - Light sensitivity
  - MSDS
  - Need for stabilizers, or other components to help efficacy or activity

The screening process is really the beginning of the development report that will be used in determining the parameters that are used in production and thus the process validation protocol (Refer to

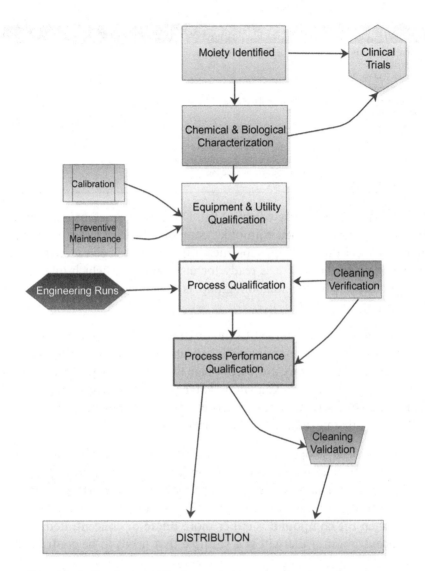

Figure 7.1 General flow from discovery to distribution.

Chapter 8: The Process Validation Protocol—PPQ). Results from the screening provide information about effectiveness, concentration needed, solubility, availability to the cells, and more. Thus, the process definition begins with the research department.

As the process (production of larger quantities of the active compound) is scaled up and further developed, several items need to be monitored and recorded. The active moiety is now referred to as the

Table 7.1 Basic Parameters to Monitor

- Temperature(s) used in production—each step of the process
- Flow rates
- Content uniformity requirements
- Pressure requirements
- Concentrations of all materials added to the process
- Times of additions
- Order of additions
- Rates of reactions
- Completeness of reactions and the time it takes to complete
- Environmental conditions—for example, exposure to light, oxygen, etc.
- Safety factors—operator and product safety in handling
- Intermediates formed during production

Active Pharmaceutical Ingredient (API). During the development workup the API is often combined with other components (excipients) or inactive ingredients to form the drug substance or product (it is considered a drug substance up to the time it is ready for distribution, at which time it is a drug product). The formulation group is generally responsible for this latter activity.

As the materials are added to the mixture to make the drug product, care must be taken to monitor each operation (addition, mixing, granulation, etc.). These items are used when the validation protocol is prepared and the process is validated. Table 7.1 is a short list of some of the items to be monitored during process development (for clinical trials) as they provide information on the variables of the process itself.

The chemical properties are determined, the growth or separation conditions are determined, and the conditions to increase its pharmacologic activity (if any) are also determined. As this work is going on, the variations are noted and recorded. For example, the best activity is found when the compound is either more dilute or concentrated. Thus, the concentration of the API is a variable that needs to be controlled.

In other words, as the process is being developed and scaled up, all chemical and physical parameters need to be monitored and recorded. The development group will also be looking at events or conditions that cause the API to act "differently" as far as expected activity on the cells or test animals. This is now the start of determining the variables of activity. This also leads to the identification of "critical" and "noncritical" steps and operations. That is, your Critical Process Parameters (CPP) and Critical Quality Attributes (CQA).

As discussed above, during scale up the development group records variations that occur to the API during production. As variations are noted, steps are taken to control that variable. For example, using the statin example above; if development finds that the activity of the API falls considerably when the batch is heated over 80°C, the group has now determined that it must be kept below that temperature during production—thus a CPP is born.

The question then becomes "Why is the temperature control critical at that stage?" To answer this question the API is sent back to the research group. They do a study and try to resolve this issue. The understanding of the variations and their causes is a big part of the new FDA 2011 Process Validation Guideline requirements.[3] In any case, the development group has it under control and has it recorded as a CPP.

RISK ASSESSMENT

Yet another major aspect of developing the product and the process is a risk analysis. The FDA guidance for process validation stresses the use of risk management for the development of the process validation program. The FDA uses the ICH Q9[4] guideline as the main basis for developing a risk management program. ICH Q9 addresses how risk should be evaluated and handled (Fig. 7.2). It presents a program to assure that the risk has been fully evaluated and it has been communicated to all workers. It then goes further in addressing a review on a regular basis to determine if the risk is still a present threat over time.

The risk referred to, in this case, is the risk to the patient. But this risk may come from many places. There are several possible sources of risk and thus error during production. As seen below, each area has its own possible source of error and thus it becomes a risk to the patient. It must be determined which risk or possible error poses a substantial risk and this needs to be corrected or prevented from occurring. Several organizations have published risk management programs (eg, ISPE Risk-Mapp) to address these risk areas. Table 7.2 below outlines some of the general risk types that need to be considered.

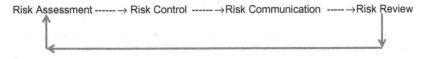

Figure 7.2 ICH Q9 approach. Source: ICH Q9.[7]

Table 7.2 General Types of Risk

- Equipment
  - Machine failures
  - Cleaning
  - Setup issues
- Ingredients
  - API
  - Excipients
- People
  - Operator skills
  - Maintenance
  - Cleaning
- Understanding
  - Training

Table 7.3 Points to Consider in Determining Risk

- Risk to benefits comparison
- Product availability
- Quality systems
- Product development knowledge
- Probability and severity of hazard
- Acceptable levels of risk
- Patient population (age, condition)
- Number of products made at a given site
- Exposure (volume of products in commerce)
- Dosage form and rout of administration
- Number of process steps

With the above list of general risks one needs to start determining the outcome of each if the risk were to present itself. Table 7.3 shows some points to consider when determining if a risk is real, and how to address the risk. Some references on risk analysis, and risk handling are found (PAT[5] (Process Analytical Technology), ICH[6] [Q8, Q9, Q10], QSIT[7] (Quality Systems Inspections Technique), The Quality System Approach (GMPs for the 21st Century)[8]).

Evaluating the level of risk is accomplished in one of several ways:

- **FTA** (Fault Tree Analysis)
- **FMEA** (Failure Mode Effect Analysis)
- **FMECA** (Failure Mode, Effect and Criticality Analysis)
- **HACCP** (Hazard Analysis Critical Control Points)

Most of the analysis performed in pharmaceuticals is by the FMEA approach. An example of this is seen in Figs. 7.3 and 7.4.

OWNER	ITEM	DETECTABILITY	OCCURRENCE	SEVERITY	RPN
Engineering	Mixer				
	Runs Slow	4	1	5	20
	Runs Fast	4	1	5	20
	Intermitent Fast & Slow	2	2	5	20
	Product Level Low	5	3	5	75
	Product Level High	4	3	5	60
	Power loss	5	1	1	5
					0
Compounding	API				
	High trace metals	2	3	4	24
	Clumped	4	3	3	36
	Smell	5	1	2	10
	Combined lots	5	2	3	30
	Combined different suppliers	1	2	3	6
	Color incorrect	2	3	4	24
	Particle distribution low	3	4	5	60
	Particle distribution high	3	4	5	60
					0
Operations	Batch Record				
	Missing a page	4	2	5	40
	Not approved completely	4	1	5	20
	Old version	5	2	5	50

Rate from 1 to 5			
1	Easy to Spot	Infrequent	Not Important
2			
3	Average	Average	Average
4			
5	Hard to Spot	Often	Very Sever

Figure 7.3 Example of an FMEA.

OWNER	ITEM	DETECTABILITY	OCCURRENCE	SEVERITY	RPN
Engineering	Power loss	5	1	1	5
Compounding	Combined different suppliers	1	2	3	6
Compounding	Smell	5	1	2	10
Engineering	Runs Slow	4	1	5	20
Engineering	Runs Fast	4	1	5	20
Engineering	Intermittent Fast & Slow	2	2	5	20
Operations	Not approved completely	4	1	5	20
Compounding	High trace metals	2	3	4	24
Compounding	Color incorrect	2	3	4	24
Compounding	Combined lots	5	2	3	30
Compounding	Clumped	4	3	3	36
Operations	Missing a page	4	2	5	40
Operations	Old version	5	2	5	50
Engineering	Product Level High	4	3	5	60
Compounding	Particle distribution low	3	4	5	60
Compounding	Particle distribution high	3	4	5	60
Engineering	Product Level Low	5	3	5	75

Figure 7.4 FMEA sorted by RPN.

According to ASQ[9] the FMEA is used:

- When a process, product, or service is being designed or redesigned
- When an existing process, product, or service is being applied in a new way
- Before developing control plans for a new or modified process
- When improvement goals are planned for an existing process, product, or service
- When analyzing failures of an existing process, product, or service
- Periodically throughout the life of the process, product, or service

PROCESS PARAMETERS

Every process needs limits. As discussed below, the process limits are considered critical or noncritical. These are predicated on both the critical and noncritical parameters of the process being met (Fig. 7.5). As the Webster dictionary defines critical[10,11]

> **CRITICAL** a: of, relating to, or being a turning point or specially important juncture <a critical phase>: as (1) : relating to or being the stage of a disease at which an abrupt change for better or worse may be expected; also : being or relating to an illness or condition involving danger of death <critical care> <a patient listed in critical condition> (2) : **relating to or being a state in which or a measurement or point at which some quality, property, or phenomenon suffers a definite change** <critical temperature>
> b : crucial, decisive <a critical test>
> c : indispensable, vital ... <a component critical to the operation of a machine>

Note the definition in (2) above. This is what is referred to as a critical process parameter. If the parameter changes then a CQA will change and the process will be different than allowed for in the criteria. Table 7.4 Shows some examples of CPPs and CQAs.

Thus, a noncritical step or operation is one that is not vital or important to the production of the product but is needed to further the process. For example, if the mixing time is considered a noncritical step in the process then the mixing parameter can be set for a reasonable time, for example, 3–5 min. This allows the product to be mixed but does not delay the remaining steps of the process.

From these definitions it is clear that one must control, at a minimum, the critical process step or operation. As stated earlier, to

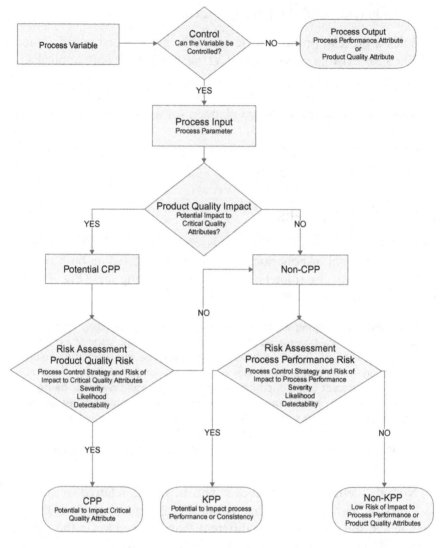

Figure 7.5 Decision tree for designating parameter criticality. Source: PDA TR60.

succeed at process validation the variables of the process need to be understood and controlled. Those steps or operations that are considered critical, that is, absolutely necessary for the successful formation of the product as defined in research and development, are the CPPs. These CPPs lead to CQAs that must be met in order to have a reproducible process and one that is in control.

Table 7.4 Some CPPs and CQAs
Examples of CPPs
• Agitation speed • Cooling/heating rate • Flow rate • Hold time • Mixing speed • Mixing time • Order of addition • Pressure • Process duration • Reynolds number • Temperature • Time (each step) • Vacuum
Examples of CQAs
• Color • Dissolution • Hardness • pH • Sterility • Temperature • Viscosity

Control of the CPPs and thus the CQAs assures that the product meets all necessary chemical and physical attributes to function as intended. It is important to get the critical and noncritical parameters from the research or development groups in writing (ie, a development report) prior to writing the validation protocol.

SETTING PROCESS LIMITS

Once the basic process of making the drug product has been developed, an analysis of the places and chances of an error is evaluated, and remediation steps are developed (or have been taken), the development group sets the process limits. As pointed out earlier in the example of the statins, going over 80°C is where a process limit has been reached. The limits that need to be set are:

- Edge of Failure (EOF)—this is where 50% of the time the product meets all process and release criteria
- Control Limits (CL) (usually also the Validation Limits)—these are maximum boundaries in which the product meets all specifications. Tighter than EOF values
- Proven Acceptable Range (PAR)—this range is established during the validation process. Validation usually uses the Upper and Lower

control limits as the limits for the PAR. Range within which acceptable material is produced. Typically used in Regulatory filing
- Normal Operating Range (NOR)—these are the conditions that the production is run at under normal conditions—all criteria are met. Tighter ranges than the Control Limits are used for routine production to ensure consistency. Must account for plant capabilities
- Target (T)—this is the middle of the normal operation range. Operators use this as the starting set point for production

A good development report will include all of these boundaries (except the PAR which needs additional proof during process validation). The limits are set according to meeting both physical and chemical characteristics of the product. Keep in mind that every product is individual, even in a family of products. Because of this if a matrix approach is used for a set of similar products or for a family of products (those products having the same ingredients but differ with the concentrations) care must be taken to cover the "worst" case conditions. These are conditions that are the hardest to control (eg, lowest weight of the API).

In addition to the PAR, NOR, and EOF limits (Fig. 7.6), one also has to set alert and action limits (alarm levels) for the process. The alert limit is the level that when reached informs the operators that the process is tending to run either higher or lower than expected. The operation should be carefully monitored so as to keep all parameters within their control points. This is a point at which the operation needs

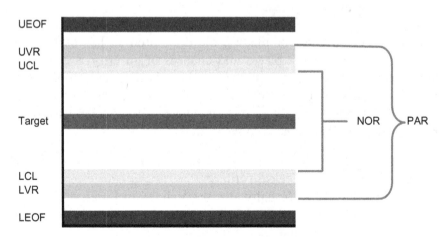

Figure 7.6 Setting parameters.

to be more carefully monitored. The action limit is the level that when reached tells the operators that the system is close to not working within specifications. The process should be stopped and an evaluation made as to what and why the action limit has been reached. Both the alert and action limits should be set within the NOR range established.

NEXT STEPS

Once the Equipment and Utility Qualificationprocess has been planned. R&D has determined the parameters, and scale up is in the process of being implemented, there are still items that need to be completed prior to the actual validation itself. The most important of these is performing a Process Qualification (PQ) during development of the process and/or during scale up. This PQ (this may in some cases be considered Engineering Runs) is not the Process Performance Qualification or PPQ that is the process validation. This PQ is to run the process in its entirety and to make sure that all parameters work together. During development, as with the qualification of the process equipment, each step of the process is tested individually. In the case of equipment qualification the Installation Qualification (IQ) and Operational Qualification (OQ) tests are all stand-alone pieces of equipment (see Chapter 5: Basic Equipment and Utility Qualification).

During the PQ testing adjustments can be made to the process, and recorded as was done during commissioning for the equipment. The equipment cannot be changed without a formal change control; however, at the stage of the PQ the system has not been validated for the process so changes are allowed (within reason, that being within the specifications previously established) as long as there is a good documentation trail. A well-run process PQ is important to the obtaining a complete and trouble free.

Thus, once the production has been developed, risk analyzed (more risks can be added during production if necessary), the APIs' conditions established, the CPPs established, and the PQ and/or engineering runs performed, the PPQ can be prepared and the process validation program can continue.

NOTES

1. Medicinal chemistry is that group that selects or synthesizes the chemical to be screened by the research group. The research department itself often performs this task.

2. Guidance for Industry Process Validation: General Principles and Practices, FDA January 2011.

3. Albers-Schönberg, G., Joshua, H., Lopez, M.B., Hensens, O.D., Springer, J.P., Chen, J., Ostrove, S., Hoffman, C.H., Alberts, A.W., Patchett, A.A., Dihydromevinolin, a potent hypocholesterolemic metabolite produced by *Aspergillus terreus*. J Antibiot (Tokyo). 1981 May 34(5):507–12.

4. ICH Guidance for Industry: Q9 Quality Risk Management, FDA, Jun. 2006 ICH.

5. Guidance for Industry: PAT—A Framework for Innovative Pharmaceutical Development, Manufacturing and Quality Assurance, FDA, Sep. 2004.

6. Guidance for Industry; Q10 Pharmaceutical Quality Systems Q10, FDA, Apr. 2009 ICH; Guidance for Industry: Q9 Quality Risk Management, FDA, Jun. 2006 ICH.

7. Guide to the Inspection of Quality Systems, FDA, Aug. 1999.

8. Pharmaceutical CGMPs for the 21st Century—A Risk-Based Approach Final Report; FDA, Sept. 2004.

9. ASQ web site.

10. Technical Report No. 60, PDA, Process Validation: A Life Cycle Approach, 2013, p. 22—with permission.

11. Merriam–Webster on line dictionary—http://www.merriam-webster.com/dictionary/critical.

CHAPTER 8

The Process Validation Protocol—PPQ

INTRODUCTION

The process validation protocol is relatively easy to prepare **IF** all of the characterizations and work up of the process has been completed in Stage I. By the time the process performance protocol (PPQ) is to be written the following items should have been prepared and completed (approved and signed as necessary):

- The Validation Master Plan
- All Process Equipment to be used in the process has been qualified
- All Process utilities to be used have been at least commissioned and/or qualified
- Computer systems and Automation controls are qualified/validated
- The process has been fully worked out and the sources of variation have been identified
- All CPPs (Critical Process Parameters) and CQAs (Critical Quality Attributes) have been identified[1]
- Scale up has been completed (PPQ should be run at full production scale and in the production equipment)
- The Master Batch Record has been prepared
- Engineering Studies have been performed as necessary

But obviously there is more to the program than just determining the variables, the CPPs, and the CQAs. Stage II, as discussed in the 2011 Process Validation guideline from the US Food and Drug Administration (FDA), follows Stage I activity and builds on it.

The process validation protocol is a document like any other prospective protocol, that is, a test plan with predetermined acceptance criteria. The primary basis for the protocol is the batch record since you are trying to prove that the process is reproducible and under control. The number of batches run will depend on the product, how well the development work was done, and of course the results of the testing in the protocol.

How to Validate a Pharmaceutical Process. DOI: http://dx.doi.org/10.1016/B978-0-12-804148-2.00008-1

Although it has been "industry standard" that one needs three consecutive successful batches to prove the validated or compliant state of the process, this is not true today. As found in both the 1987 and 2011 Process Validation guidelines the FDA states that a sufficient number of batches will be run. In addition, the 2011 guideline states that there will be continued process verification (CPV) after the process has been deemed compliant (Stage III). This means that continued checking of process parameters is needed to demonstrate control. In other words, process validation is really never complete.

SETTING PROTOCOL TEST RANGES

In writing the process validation protocol (now referred to as the Process Performance Qualification or PPQ) the starting point should be a list of all of the CPPs and CQAs as found in the development reports (Stage I). The ranges tested should also be noted, as this will be a big factor in how many and what type of process runs will be made. As discussed in Chapter 7, "Process Development," on process development, determining the ranges that will yield a consistent product is the job of Stage I.

There are several ranges that need to be fully addressed in a complete process validation program. Setting and developing these were discussed in Chapter 7, "Process Development." These ranges are (refer to Figs. 8.1 and 8.2):

- Target
- Upper and Lower Proven Acceptable Range (Upper and Lower Control or Validation Range)
- Upper and Lower Normal Operating Range
- Upper and Lower Edge of Failure

Notice in Fig. 8.1 the Normal Operation Range falls within the Proven Acceptable Range that falls within the Edge of Failure. The target, at the top of the pyramid is in the center of all of the ranges. Fig. 8.2 shows this graphically.

In the past it has been the practice of the industry to run three batches at what is known as the target value. Target is the middle point of all the ranges (Figs. 8.2 or 8.3). Proving the process runs correctly at the midpoint is good but only a small part of what is needed. As discussed by Chapman[2] the proven acceptable range or the validation range also needs to be clearly addressed in the protocol.

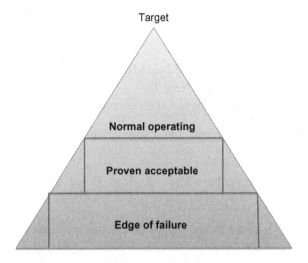

Figure 8.1 Understanding set point development.

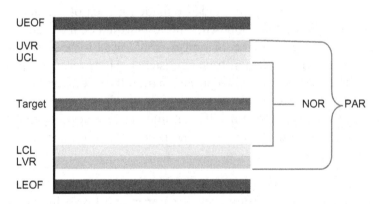

Figure 8.2 Graphical approach to set point relationships.

Let's take an example: The process is completed in four steps.

Step 1—Ingredient A is added to 100 Gal of water at 80°C ± 5°C with agitation at 250 RPM ± 10%; Total dissolution of Ingredient A; addition to be complete within 10 min.

Step 2—The solution is cooled to 25°C ± 2°C in 30 ± 5 min.

Step 3—Ingredient B is added to the cooled solution while agitating at 500 RPM ± 10%; total dissolution of Ingredient B.

Step 4—Ingredient C is slowly added to the solution so as to prevent clumping. Mixing speed is 50 ± 5 RPM; no clumping, solution has a viscosity of 500 cp.

- There are three CPPs and thus three CQAs (these are the measurable results of the CPPs)
  - CPPs
    - Temperature of mixing Ingredient A
    - Dissolution of Ingredient B
    - Addition of Ingredient C (no clumping)

With this simple scenario the ranges can be determined and the protocol set.

The Proven Acceptable range in Step 1 are temperatures within 85–75°C.

The Edge of Failure range would be outside of these temperatures.

While the Normal Operation range would be 77–82°C.

The target is 80°C.

The above determinations would be made for each of the steps in the process during Stage I development, and tests would be included for each of the CPPs. These set points or ranges would need to be tested at least three times in order to demonstrate consistency. However, if the development group has provided sufficient information the testing and proof that the process will be acceptable and repeatable for all of the ranges then the process can be run at target a sufficient number of times to complete the process validation (ie, the limits of the process have been clearly established and tested).

If on the other hand there is incomplete or insufficient information from the development group then the upper and lower limits of each range would need to be tested and demonstrate that they are real and consistent. This adds many tests to the program.

PREPARING THE PROTOCOL

In order to prepare an effective validation protocol (Fig. 8.3) you should start with the end in mind. That is, "What do you want to prove, and how do you want it demonstrated?" Table 8.1 provides a generic Table of Contents for a PPQ based on a process model (Table 8.2). Some of the elements that should be found in good process validations are:

- Sampling Plan (How, What, When, and Where samples are to be taken)
- Responsibilities

Table 8.1 Table of Contents for a PPQ Protocol (Generic)[3]
• Title/approval
• Purpose
• Scope
• Process model (Table 8.2)/description
• Equipment (process and utilities)
• CQAs, CPPs, CIPCs
• Study plan
• Batch records
• Sampling/testing plan
• Comparison to bio-batch
• Uniformity/homogeneity (APIs)
• Impurity profile comparison (APIs)
• Acceptance criteria
• Responsibilities
• Discrepancies
• References

Table 8.2 Process Model
• Process description and process flow diagrams
• Discuss each unit operation in relation to the equipment and utilities used
• Outline critical process parameters, critical in-process controls, and critical quality attributes
• Describe manufacturing instructions, raw materials, and relevant procedures

- Repeatability—all results
- Robustness
- Operator to Operator Consistency
- Controlled—use of control charts (see chapter: Stage III—Collection and Evaluating Production Data)
- All CPPs and CIPC are tested
- All CQAs are met

Tests in the PPQ are based on the production batch record. Normally the product will be made according to the batch record (at target), however, during validation extra samples (both in time and quantity) need to be taken and stress conditions need to be used. Again, if development has documentation that the product can be run at various speeds, temperatures, mixing times, etc. then the PPQ is simpler. It is primarily run at target and one or two other conditions. These conditions should constitute the "worst" case conditions that one would expect to encounter during operation (eg, lowest speed and highest temperature). Worst case is not to make the product or production fail.

In demonstrating that the process is reproducible and in control (also see Chapter 10: Stage III—Collection and Evaluating Production Data), there are many items in the process pathway that need to be

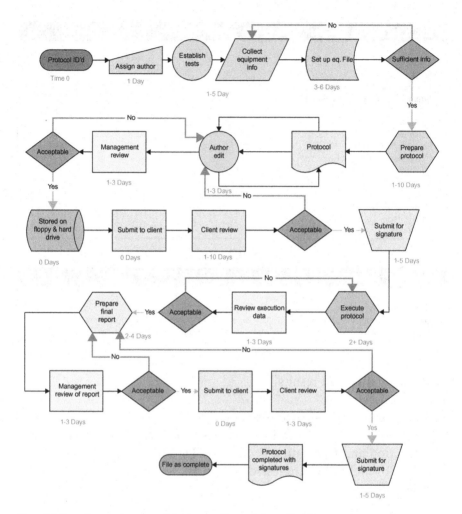

Figure 8.3 General approach to protocol development. Source: Informa Healthcare.

verified other than that it remains within the set control limits. For example, it may also include the impurities at different steps of the process (need to establish an impurity profile) and/or content uniformity. Items like this are general and may be applicable to most if not all products. Table 8.3 shows some measurable parameters (CQAs) for Tablets, Creams, Ointments and Liquid products.

Table 8.4 lists some of the items, not necessarily directly in the process line but that can influence the final product. These (as appropriate) need to be shown to be complete or effective before the process can be

Table 8.3 Some Properties to Be Tested

Tablets	Creams	Liquids/Suspensions	Comments
Content uniformity	Content uniformity	Content uniformity	Refer to USP <905 > [a]
Dissolution	Viscosity	pH	
Hardness	pH	Color	
Friability	Color	Fill volume	
Weight	Bioburden	Bioburden	No objectionable organisms
Size	Temperature	Viscosity	
Embossing/scoring	Voids	Impurity profile	
Coating	Impurity profile		Thickness/chipping

[a] *United States Pharmacopeia; Uniformity of Dosage Units <905>, United States Pharmacopeial Convention, Inc.*

Table 8.4 Other Parameters to be Tested

- Content Uniformity
- Container Closure
- Bioburden
- Hold times (between process steps)
- Computer/Automation effectiveness (see chapter: Computers and Automated Systems)
- Labels and Printing
- Stability (at each step in the process and the final product)
- Air and other Gases Quality
- Materials of construction (particularly of the primary package since this was accounted for in the equipment qualification)
- Warehousing conditions (if temperature requirements are needed for the product)

considered validated. Each of these items need to have a separate test written in the PPQ (these are often referred to as test scripts).

As with all qualification and validation protocols it needs to be approved prior to its implementation (execution). Upon completion of all tests a close out review needs to be performed and a final report prepared.

EXECUTING THE PROTOCOL

Executing the PPQ is relatively easy, as seen in Fig. 8.4. The protocol should be written, as the process would produce the product. Scale up activity has already taken place.[4,5] But before the execution starts there are several things that either should be reviewed or checked. These are:

- Review of the protocol to be sure that the correct revision is in use, so that when you start the execution you know what is needed for the testing and sampling (eg, test instruments, sample vials, etc.),

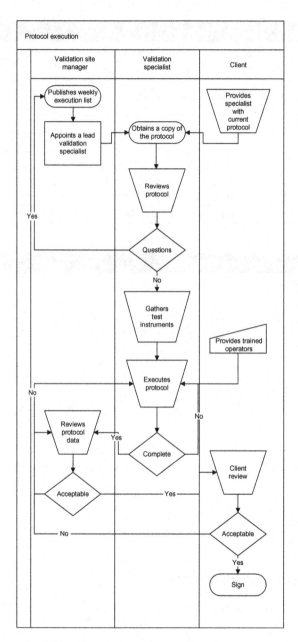

Figure 8.4 Flow plan for protocol execution.

and that you are familiar with the test(s) to be run (ie, you know how to perform the test)
- Are there sufficient sample containers of the correct type and size (volume)?
- Is the lab ready to test or store the extra samples due to the extra testing and sampling?
- Verify safety precautions. For example, is a lock out tag out protocol necessary?
- Be sure that the trained equipment operators are available for the test(s)
- All units on the process line are calibrated
- All test instruments are calibrated

Samples need to be taken from the production line at intervals that will allow a sufficient statistical[6] evaluation of the results. Each of the CPPs are tested, thus samples for each of the CQAs need to be taken several times during the run. Under normal operating conditions samples are taken at the beginning, middle, and end of each run. However, during validation executions samples need to be taken more frequently (eg, every hour).

Because of the extra samples needed during PPQ execution the QC lab or the contract lab to which the samples are to be sent for analysis must be prepared for the extra load. This includes not just the testing of the samples but also storage of the samples as necessary.

Sampling Plans[7]
There is no single approach to determining the appropriate sampling plan; however, it must be scientifically accurate to provide valid results of the testing. Plan design should include a statistician or at least some-one well versed in statistical methods. Designing a sampling plan that has the appropriate resolution to describe the process variability is an important part of building confidence in the process. Whichever approach is selected it must have a clearly defined rationale behind it. There is no right or wrong answer, but whatever sampling plan is developed must be defensible based upon the level of resolution necessary to see variation in the process as well as being statistically accurate. Thus, a large number of samples are taken at short intervals during production.

Recording the Results
As with any protocol execution the results need to be recorded using Good Documentation Practices (GDP). Recording of numbers is very

important and should follow corporate SOPs (Standard Operating Procedures) on rounding, truncation, and use of significant figures. All original data **must** be retained. Copying over of results so that the document looks neat is often a cause for transcription errors and more.

The Validation Report

When the execution is complete, that is the specified number of runs have been made and all of the samples collected and tested, the data entered, lab results are complete and confirmed as correct (ie, all calculations have been verified) the validation final report can be prepared. In addition, all deviations (see chapter: Dealing With Deviations) have been logged and the appropriate investigation executed. Remember, the protocol cannot be closed while any deviation is open. The report should follow the company SOP on validation reports and should contain the following:

- Summary of all data, preferably in table format
- A table listing all tests performed and their results—summary with an indication of Pass or Fail
  - If a test failed reference to the corrective action, retesting, and rationale should be provided
- A valid conclusion—it is recommended that the first sentence or paragraph state that the validation is (or is not) successful.
- The report can be attached to the protocol or a stand-alone document.

NOTES

1. Note: Stage III is Continued Process Verification—this allows one to add or delete CPPs and/ or CQAs based on production. This will be discussed in Chapter 10, "Stage III—Collection and Evaluating Production Data."

2. Chapman, K.: The PAR Approach to Process Validation. Pharmaceutical Technology 8(12), 22–36, 1984.

3. Ostrove, S.: Qualification and Change Control. In: Agalloco, J., Carlton, F., editors, Validation of Pharmaceutical Processes, 3rd Ed.; New York: Informa Healthcare USA, 2008, Chapter 9, pp. 129–145.

4. Note: It is sometimes possible to execute the validation runs during the scale up phase of the program. However, it is recommended that the scale used be approximately 75% of production. Full production scale is preferred.

5. Ostrove, S.: Scale-up and Process Validation. In: Levine, M., editor, Pharmaceutical Process Scale-up. New York: Informa Healthcare USA, 2011, Chapter 4, pp. 109–116.

6. ISO Standard 2859.

7. WHO Guidelines for Sampling of Pharmaceutical Products and Related Materials, WHO Technical Report Series No. 929, 2005.

CHAPTER *9*

Dealing With Deviations

Generally there are two types of exceptions or deviations that are often used in pharmaceutical manufacturing[1]

- Deficiencies—a result not meeting the expected result or condition. These do not impact or adversely affect the unit's use
- Deviation—a failure of the unit to meet its predetermined acceptance criteria that may affect its use.

These are usually just grouped into the term "deviation"[2] or "exceptions" for sake of clarity in the protocol (this chapter will use the generic term "deviation"). However, a deficiency is more serious since it may affect the process due to a "fault" in the design or construction of the equipment. For example, if the acceptance criterion is "unit is red" and the color is blue, this is a deficiency, while a deviation would be having two switches or tanks when the design calls for three.

As well as you plan and execute the validation work there is always a possibility that something will go wrong.[3] Even during commercial production things can go wrong. In a compliant system any time an operation or function does not meet the acceptance criteria established for that operation or function a deviation needs to be logged and an investigation needs to be performed. There are four major areas in which an error can occur:

- Errors made during Qualification (equipment/systems)
- Errors made during Validation (process errors or execution errors)
- Errors made in production (compounding or other batch errors)
- Errors made in the Laboratory (QC function/testing—eg, OOS (Out of Specification))

Each of these areas has its own way of determining what went wrong and how to fix it. All errors need to be recorded (and logged) and to have an investigation performed. The first case, occurring during

How to Validate a Pharmaceutical Process. DOI: http://dx.doi.org/10.1016/B978-0-12-804148-2.00009-3

equipment qualification is usually handled at a "lower" level of severity. This is because the error is usually easily fixed. By this I mean that engineering or the development group can rectify the error.

- For example, a valve is installed in the wrong place or is positioned backwards (check valves). The engineering group will review the drawing and the valve in question. They will then determine if a change needs to be made. An investigation is necessary. But here the investigation is by the engineering group.
- Another example that can occur during the Operational Qualification (OQ) is an incorrect speed or flow rate attained. Here, not only would the engineering group be involved in determining the cause, but the product development group as well. For it may be that even though the flow or speed was not obtained as specified, it may not impact the products production—for example, the process needs to have a mixing rate at 100 RPM ± 10%, yet the OQ test specified that the motor would run up to 300 RPM ± 10%. During the test it was found that the motor reached 269 RPM. Thus, it was close but failed its acceptance criteria. It would be determined that the motor was adequate for the process (ie, it meets the 100 RPM ± 10% conditions). In this case both engineering and development were involved.

In dealing with a deviation that occurs during process validation or during production a different approach is needed. Once a deviation has been noted in these cases several things need to take place. The first of these is to determine the level of the deviation. There are two levels of deviations based on the risk to the patient. Thus, a deviation can be critical or noncritical. A critical deviation is one in which the product may be or actually is compromised. In determining the level of deviation the following assessments, include but not limited to, need to be made:

- Effect on the product
- Effect on the documentation (Protocol, SOPs, batch)
- The design (drawings, system documents)
- User requirements, Engineering requirements
- Is it systemic or a one time event?

A noncritical deviation can result in an unexpected result, a misunderstanding of the requirements, or a change in procedure that has not yet gone through the change control process. A noncritical deviation does not affect the product or system integrity. One of the most common noncritical deviations is known as a "protocol generation error (PGE)." In this case an incorrect value or some other error in the preparation of the protocol occurs. When a PGE is found the validation specialist must go back to engineering or the development group in order to determine if what is in the protocol is real or an entry mistake. This can occur if the protocol is written prior to the issuing of the as-built drawings or vendor modifications. Examples of noncritical deviations are:

- Incorrect make or model number for a piece of process equipment or utility
- Incorrect specification for the unit being tested—for example, temperature was specified for an office area and changed to a process area
- Inability to read a serial number on the equipment (valve)
- Incorrect room numbering in the protocol
- Power failure during a validation test that is not due to a process operation, for example, lightning with no emergency power system

As stated previously, a critical deviation is one in which the product is or may be adversely affected. Some examples of these are:

- Failure to meet an in-process acceptance criteria
- Failure to meet a release criteria—for example, incorrect volume or weight
- Machine failure due to a process function—for example, incorrect adjustment or settings
- Valve incorrectly positioned—for example, a check valve installed incorrectly
- Data integrity error—computer or other

Fig. 9.1[4] provides a basic flow chart for determining the level of the deviation. Following the determination of the deviation level, the next step is to document the error. If the error occurred during protocol execution the event should be recorded in the deviation section of the protocol. If the error occurred during commercial production a separate log and record needs to be maintained (eg, Trackwise). In addition, the batch record needs to have the deviation recorded and the results of the investigation noted.

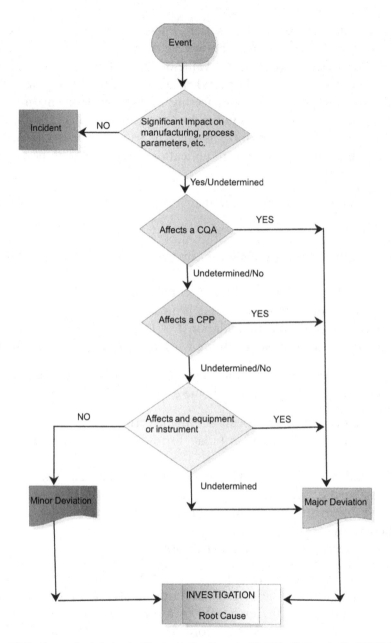

Figure 9.1 Decision tree for deviation classification. Source: From the World Health Organization (WHO).[4]

The step following the investigation is to determine if a corrective action and/or a preventative action (CAPA) are needed. Once the need for a CAPA has been determined the event can be closed.

THE INVESTIGATION[5]

Now that the type and extent of the deviation has been determined the event needs to be investigated. In both type of deviations the investigation for the real reason for the error needs to be determined, that is, the root cause.[6] The FDA looks at the investigation very carefully.[7] It is not sufficient to say that the operator, or analyst in the laboratory made the error. The root cause for the error needs to be established. If, after careful review of relevant facts there is no "root cause" apparent then the next best is the most likely cause. In performing an investigation[8] the following need to be considered:

- What really happened? (The problem needs to be clearly defined)
- Who was involved (those working the line at the time)
  - Associated personnel—those bringing in the equipment (setup) or the materials for production
  - Cleaning or maintenance personnel
  - Guests
- Other events
  - May not seem related
    - Last product made on the line—line clearance
    - Similar event(s) on other production lines
    - Similar events with other similar equipment
  - Other process lines or equipment? that is, not similar equipment but similar event(s)
- Other lots affected?
- Natural occurrences—for example, power outage due to storm
- Other products affected either at the same time or recent past?

The investigation requires a team approach since different departments may have differing ideas and see things a little differently. You shouldn't expect that the investigation will be a short event. In many cases it takes weeks or even months to reach the true root cause of the deviation.

NOTES

1. There are many definitions and terms used for "errors" and other nonconformances in production, these terms are used here as an illustration.

2. Title 21 CFR 211.100, FDA, 2015.

3. O'Keeffe, G.: Validation Deviations—An Important Part of any Validation Project, on www. askaboutgmp.com, May 2013.

4. Deviation Handling and Quality Risk Management, World Health Organization, p. 9, Jul. 2013.

5. Title 21 CFR 211.180.

6. Anderson, B., Fagerhaug, T.: Root Cause Analysis Simplified Tools and Techniques, Ed. 2, ASQ Quality Press, Milwaukee, WI, 2006.

7. Smith, P., Elder, D.: Regulation and Compliance: Deviation Investigations, PharmTech 36(4), 2012.

8. Anonymous, The Top Ten Reasons the Deviation Investigation System Fails, QA Pharm, Jan. 2011 on http://www.mbtmag.com/article/2011/01/top-10-reasons-deviation-investigation-system-fails

Stage III—Continued Process Verification

CHAPTER 10

Stage III—Collection and Evaluating Production Data

GENERAL APPROACH

To start Stage III or Continued Process Verification (CPV)[1] the company must have a written plan. Most existing products that have already been validated are at least partly in compliance with this stage of process validation since each product must have an annual review that includes monitoring of the process parameters and continuity of consistency in product attributes. However, now each batch needs to be evaluated for trends, adherence to process controls, and general reliability of the safety of the product (ie, CPV). According to the US Food and Drug Administration (FDA) this means that even after the process is considered validated the manufacturer needs to demonstrate assurance that the process is capable of maintaining a state of control, that is, validation or compliance. According to 21 CFR 211.180(e) there must be a program that reviews and analyzes data collected during production. This program as with all other programs needs to be written, reviewed on a regular basis, and practiced.

The current expectation of the FDA is that the CPV will include more information than the Annual Product Review (APRs). It is intended to detect unplanned departures from the design of the process. While the APRs provide information about production (eg, number of batches produced, number of batches accepted of rejected, complaints, etc.) the current thinking is that there needs to be a demonstration of full process control, that is, control of the Critical Process Parameters (CPPs) and Critical Quality Attributes (CQAs). Each batch should be reviewed for compliance to its specifications. One way of approaching this is the use of control charts for each of the CPP/CQAs (Fig. 10.1).[2] In addition, action limits need to be established so that if there is a deviation from the expected results a correction can be made before the process is out of control or a batch needs to be rejected for not meeting all acceptance criteria. If a CQA appears over or under its acceptance

How to Validate a Pharmaceutical Process. DOI: http://dx.doi.org/10.1016/B978-0-12-804148-2.00010-X

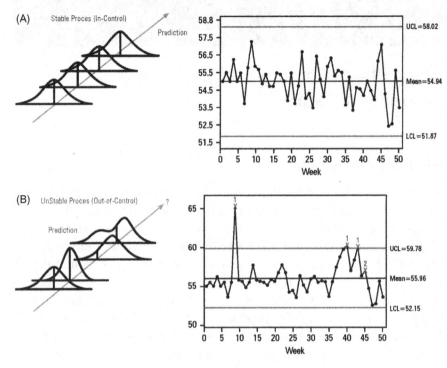

Figure 10.1 (A) Examples of a stable process (statistically in control). (B) Examples of an unstable process (statistically out of control). Source: PDA TR59.[5]

criteria a correction needs to be made. However, prior to implementing any correction other groups (not just production/operations) need to be consulted (eg, QA, development, validation, regulatory) so that the adjustment in the process maintains its compliant status. In other words, it is part of the change control program.

The FDA mentions that the performance review should include statistical analysis of the data.[3] Thus, a statistician (or at least someone competent in statistics) needs to be on the review team. The program should include trending (see Figure 10.1) so that individual events do not cause "over reaction" or over corrections. There are many statistical approaches possible to adequately do this analysis.[4]

An area that is often overlooked during the CPV review during Stage III is that of the facility. The equipment and utilities also must be kept not only operational within the specifications set for the process but they must be included in the continuous improvement program. The process utilities and equipment need to be included in a preventive maintenance program (PM) as well as a calibration program (discussed in Chapter 5).

Another aspect of the CPV program is to enable continuous improvement to the process. This must be done within the change control system. Keep in mind that not all changes determined to be a continuous process improvement can be made without informing the FDA. As discussed in Chapter 3, "The Validation Life Cycle and Change Control," prior to implementation the FDA must approve any changes considered to be "major" changes.

LEGACY PRODUCTS

This book until now has been describing process validation for "new" products, that is, products that have reached the Process Performance Qualification (PPQ) stage after the promulgation of the 2011 FDA guideline. However, there are many products currently on the market that were validated under the old, 1987, guideline. The FDA expects that the new guideline will be applied to all products. However, the language in the Guidance such as "can" and "would likely begin" in the section on Legacy products, leaves the door open for pointing out that it is not strictly required. By performing a full review of existing data, the rationale for the parameters specified, and the annual reports *may* satisfy current requirements without any further developmental work.

In any case, in order to bring existing products into compliance with the new guideline requirements manufacturers need to do a thorough review of the information and results of past validation efforts. In other words, they need to start with a complete Stage III review. Upon completion of this review, they may find that the existing approach satisfies the current guideline and the process remains in compliance. However, they are more likely to find that the development information is lacking (ie, Stage I needs to be redone or improved).

A good starting point for this Stage III review is the Annual Product Review (APR). According to 21 CFR 211.180 the APR review should include all batches manufactured in the last 12 months. Generally the review of the batches is for release specifications only and not each CQA. In addition, the APR review includes a review of complaints on each batch, a review of the PM program, and a review of other "fixes" that occurred during the 12-month period. What needs to be added is a review of the development work that was done for the product that led to the process validation.

As part of the review process, production capability (C_p and C_{pk}), needs to be calculated (formulas below) in order to demonstrate that the manufacturing of the product is consistently produced according to preapproved specifications. In addition, the process performance over time (P_p and P_{pk}) will need to be evaluated. These will be discussed further later in this chapter.

In order to bring current processes into line with the current guideline the following steps can be taken.

1. Where and when possible collect the development data for each product
   a. Review the scientific literature related to and any other available information on the process
      i. Has anything changed?
         1. What were the previous process steps?
         2. Has there been any drift or trend during production over time—if so this needs to be fully evaluated
      ii. Any improvements in the chemistry?
   b. Perform additional testing where the original work is felt to be weak of incomplete
2. Reevaluate the CPPs and CQAs
   a. Are they still critical?
   b. Are they all necessary?
   c. Are any other steps now found to be "critical"?
3. Any change made to the process should be fully developed and tested prior to implementation regardless of how minor it is considered. For example:
   a. Line speed adjustments even within "validated ranges"
   b. Cleaning conditions
4. Be sure to follow all corporate change control and documentation procedures

Once you have completed the evaluation of the process you can begin implementation of the items identified. This probably will not require a full validation or revalidation of the process. As changes to the process are made, document (Change Control)

- The reason for the change
- How the change is to be implemented
- The chemical and physical properties affected by the change

Some additional testing to demonstrate bioequivalence and bio-availability may also be necessary. However, this is unlikely since the process has already been fully validated. It is the documentation that is usually lacking, not the physical testing.

Gaps in Stage I, process design data, possibly due to the age of the product or the process was obtained from other pharmaceutical companies, present significant risks to collecting additional data.

STAGE III—CONTINUED PROCESS VERIFICATION (CPV)

The CPV program involves ongoing management of the process to provide continual assurance that it remains in a state of control (validated state). This is managed through the traditional practices of Change Control, Process Metrics, Trend Analysis, and Annual Product Reviews.

1. Change Control—(Discussed in Chapter 3: "The Validation Life Cycle and Change Control") Formal Change Control procedures need to be followed in order to justify and document any change to the equipment or in the case of legacy products change to the validated process or system. Note that process validation is equipment-specific; hence any substitution of equipment (eg, alternate tanks or agitators) should be documented via the appropriate change control procedure
2. Process Metrics—Metrics should be employed to track process problems, equipment use time, line stoppages, etc. This metric review will give the company an oversight of how well and how efficiently the process is working. Keep in mind that while process efficiency or yields are not a Good Manufacturing Practice (GMP) nor FDA requirement, it is an indication that all CPPs and CQAs are being met and that the process in in control.
3. Trend Analysis—This makes use of the control charts discussed below. Each CQA should be tracked on a control chart and any trend evaluated. Trends may be due to things like seasonal variation in the water supply or equipment functionality. Statistical analysis should be employed in the analysis of the trends so that a correct interpretation can be made. Outliers can be identified and treated accordingly.

4. Annual Product Review—GMPs require that the quality of each product be reviewed at least once per year to assure that the process remains in control. The process of Annual Product Review is the typical means for regular confirmation of the compliant or validated state. Annual Product Reviews will be performed for each product in accordance with established Standard Operating Procedures (SOPs). The APRs will now cover all aspects of production as specified in the Process Validation Guideline and 21 CFR 211.180 and will typically include:
   a. Finished Product Results
   b. In-Process Results
   c. Stability Results
   d. Nonconformances
   e. Complaints
   f. Returns
   g. Recalls
   h. Summary of Changes
   i. Recommended Improvements or Corrective Actions
   j. Summary of trends and analysis performed under the Process Metrics activity.
   k. Conclusion regarding the state of the process
   l. Review and approval by appropriate technical, quality, and management personnel

STATISTICAL PROCESS CONTROL AND CONTROL CHARTS

Generally, the standard bell curve (Fig. 10.2[5]) is used to view the outcome of a production run. This graph of the product outcome shows the three standard deviations (σ) on each side of the mean. This gives an overall 6σ chart (Table 10.1[6]). These graphs are compiled first by collecting data from the run for each CQA (eg, tablet weight, tablet thickness, dissolution times, etc.) and produce a histogram (see Fig. 10.3[7]) of this data. The mean and standard deviation are also calculated. Each of these are plotted on a separate graph thus showing the "trend" that these parameters have taken over all of the lots produced. Using the formulas below the C_{pk}, the C_p, the P_p, and the P_{pk} can be calculated.[8]

C_p = Process Capability.

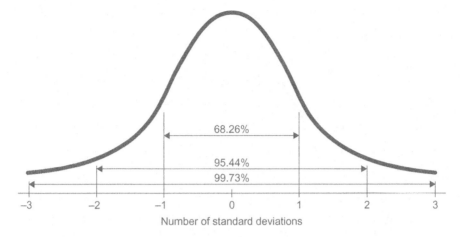

Figure 10.2 Normal distribution. Source: PDA TR-59.[5]

Table 10.1 Significance of C_p			
Value of C_p	**$C_p = 0.5$**	**$C_p = 1$**	**$C_p = 3$**
Graphical view of a process at different values of C_p	Lower limit Upper limit	Lower limit Upper limit	Lower limit Upper limit
Sigma value in the given limits	$3\sigma(\pm 1.5\sigma)$	$6\sigma(\pm 3\sigma)$	$18\sigma(\pm 9\sigma)$
Statistical number of values outside the limits	13.58%	0.27%	Really 0
Statistical number of values outside the limits	86.42%	99.73%	>99.999999%
Result	Process statistically expected to routinely make nonconforming product	Process statistically unlikely to make nonconforming product	

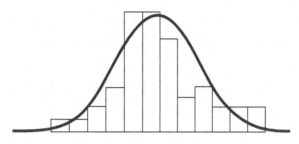

Figure 10.3 Using a histogram of a CQA to produce a normal distribution curve. Source: www.moorestream.com.[7]

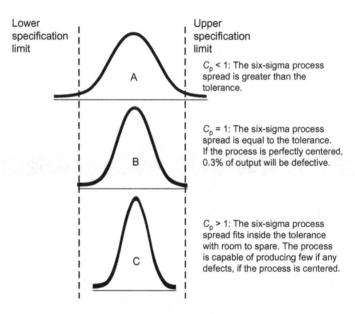

Figure 10.4 Demonstration of the meaning of C_p's related to the normal distribution. Source: www.moorestream.com.[7]

C_{pk} = Process Capability Index. This adjusts the C_p for the effect of noncentered distribution.

P_p = Process Performance.

P_{pk} = Process Performance Index. This adjusts the P_p for the effect of noncentered distribution.[7]

In looking at a graphic representation Fig. 10.4[7] shows the results of different levels of C_p. Note that with a C_p of less than 1 the production is very spread out within the set limits. While a C_p value >1 shows a very tight fit of all data points. Another way of looking at it and interpreting the results of the calculations is:

Here we are looking at the fit within a door frame (set limits)[9]

C_{pk} = 1/2 means you've crunched against the door frame

C_{pk} = 1 means you're just touching the nearest frame

C_{pk} = 2 means your width can grow 2 times before touching

C_{pk} = 3 means your width can grow 3 times before touching

Formulas for calculating C_p, C_{pk}, P_p, and P_{pk}[10]

$$\hat{\sigma} = \frac{\bar{s}}{c_4}$$

c_4 representing a statistical coefficient of correction.

$\bar{s}$ representing the mean of deviation for each rational subgroup

$$C_p = \frac{USL - LSL}{6 \times \hat{\sigma}}$$

$$C_{pk} = \min\left(\frac{USL - \mu}{3 \times \hat{\sigma}}, \frac{\mu - LSL}{3 \times \hat{\sigma}}\right)$$

$$P_{pk} = \min\left(\frac{USL - \mu}{3 \times \hat{\sigma}}, \frac{\mu - LSL}{3 \times \hat{\sigma}}\right)$$

$$P_p = \frac{USL - LSL}{6 \times s}$$

From the above discussion one can readily see the importance of incorporating and understanding the calculations and importance of the Process Capability and Process Performance calculations. The CPV program is not complete without a full analysis of the process capability and the demonstration of consistency in operation and the ability to remain "centered."

NOTES

1. Guidance for Industry Process Validation: General Principles and Practices, FDA, Jan. 2011.

2. Technical Report No. 59; Utilization of Statistical Methods for Production Monitoring, Parenteral Drug Association, 2012 (with permission).

3. Guidance for Industry Process Validation: General Principles and Practices, FDA, Jan. 2011.

4. The Book of Statistical Process Control, 2nd Ed., Cincinnati, OH, 2010, Zontec.

5. Technical Report No. 59; Utilization of Statistical Methods for Production Monitoring, Parenteral Drug Association, 2012 (with permission).

6. Ibid (with permission).

7. http://www.MoreStream.com/Knowledgecenter/toolbox/Statistical Process Control.

8. David Ruffler, Understanding how C_p and C_{pk} are Used to Ensure Quality, IsoTemp Research, Inc. Document No. 146–008, May 1996.

9. http://www.isisixsigma.com, Process Capability (C_p, C_{pk}) and Process Performance (P_p, P_{pk}) - What is the Difference?

10. The book of Statistical Process Control, 2nd Ed., Cincinnati, OH, 2010, Zontex.

Other Related Activities

CHAPTER 11

Cleaning and Facility Qualification

FACILITY DESIGN

No discussion of process validation would be complete without considering the design of the facility and the cleaning process. As specified in 21 CFR Subpart C, buildings and facilities are a major part of the Current Good Management Practice (CGMP) program. The facility must meet certain standards in order to manufacture a pharmaceutical product within its walls. The Good Manufacturing Practices (GMPs) include, for example, the size of the structure—is it large enough to safely perform all of the steps necessary to product the product? For example, the ceilings must be high enough to accommodate the removal of the tops of tanks. Other considerations found in the GMPs[1] are:

- Building location—21 CFR 211.42—so that materials and finished product can easily be moved in and out of the facility
- Lighting—21 CFR 211.44—the correct level and type (color and/or temperature) needs to be available in all work areas. For example, inspection of particles in liquid vials requires a different amount and type of light that a tablet press operation would require.
- HVAC—21 CFR 211.46—the quality of the air, the temperature and humidity, as well as viable and nonviable particles all need to be considered in designing a CGMP facility and play a big part in the process validation. The four major classifications of process rooms are:
  - Unclassified
  - ISO 8 (Class 100,000 or Class D)[2]
  - ISO 7 (Class 10,000 or Class C)
  - ISO 5 (Class 100 or Class A/B, where A is active and B is inactive)

  Examples of areas using these HVAC classifications

  Unclassified Areas
  - Warehouse
  - Offices

How to Validate a Pharmaceutical Process. DOI: http://dx.doi.org/10.1016/B978-0-12-804148-2.00011-1

- General Hallways
- Meeting Rooms

ISO 8—Class 100,000—Class D

- Compounding Rooms[3]
- General Process Operations (closed processes, initial process steps)
- In-Process storage/Staging (if storage units are closed)

ISO 7—Class 10,000—Class C

- Chemical work areas
- Filling[4]/Packaging (Solid Oral Dose, etc.)
- Clean Storage Areas

ISO 5—Class 100—Class A/B

- Aseptic Fill
- Biotechnology products (recombinant, cell-derived products)
- Clean storage areas for aseptic processes

There are other facility design criteria discussed in the Title 21 of the CFR. For example, in 21 CFR 211.48, 211.50, and 211.52 the piping, location, and slopes of both process and sanitary lines, and rest room locations are discussed.[5] These do not directly impact the process validation program, however, they must be correctly designed and installed before any process work can be started or the facility will not meet current US Food and Drug Administration (FDA) expectations.

Some additional facility qualification concerns that need to be addressed and tested prior to the process validation should include:

- Access—limit access to authorized personnel by using card readers, lock and key, etc.
- Vibration—keep all equipment running freely without stress of vibrations that can lower the life of the equipment
- Windows—caulking, etc.
- Floor/Walls/Ceiling penetrations—all should be sealed

As a last step in completing a complete and effective process validation the facility also needs to be qualified. All too often manufacturers leave this part off of their qualification program thinking that since all of the process equipment and utilities have been qualified and the process is shown to be reproducible all is finished. Table 11.1 shows some construction elements that need to be reviewed and audited prior to producing the product.

One last major consideration that needs to be included in the facility qualification program is the layout of all of the process equipment

Table 11.1 Basic Check List for Facility Qualification				
To Be Checked	Uncontrolled	ISO 8	ISO 7	ISO 5
Doors/number/types/handles	X	X	X	X
Floor—Material of Construction (MOC)-finish		X	X	X
Wall—MOC-finish		X	X	X
Ceiling—MOC-finish		X	X	X
Coving				X
Room dimensions	X	X	X	X
Lighting/type/number	X	X	X	X
Electrical/number/types	X	X	X	X
Painttype		X	X	X
Floor drains	X	X		
Pipe slope/type/welds (type and inspections)		X	X	X
Water/quality/amount/pressure	X	X	X	X
Gases	X	X	X	X
Steam	X	X	X	X
HVAC/dust/particles (viable—nonviable)	X	X	X	X
Temperature and/or humidity	X	X	X	X
Windows/vision panels		X	X	X
Vibration	X	X	X	X
Pest control—inside/outside	X	X	X	X
Air locks—before		X	X	X
Sanitary—process waste	X	X	X	X
Storage—quarantine/reject/in-process	X	X	X	X

and utilities. As stated in Chapter 5, "Basic Equipment and Utility Qualification," all equipment needs to be serviceable from all sides. This allows full operation and maintenance. As an example of where this was not accomplished, a company installed a large chromatography column in which the resin would need replacement. After installation, they discovered that the lid of the column would only open about half way. This compromised the changing of the resin and caused product failures.[6]

In general, the FDA expects that the facility floors, walls, and ceilings are made of materials that can not affect the product. That is, they are cleanable and maintained clean. As the air quality of the process room increases (ie, ISO 8 thru ISO 5) the surfaces need to be smooth, impermeable to the product and dust, and not subject to chipping or peeling so that material does not inadvertently get into the product.

INTRODUCTION TO CLEANING

Now that the process has been shown to be consistent and the Continued Process Verification (CPV) program is clearly in place and working, it is time to consider the validation of the cleaning process(s). Not only does the process equipment need to be cleaned, but also the facility. Each type of cleaning is unique and demands careful consideration. Cleaning an air handler certainly is quite different from cleaning a process reactor. However, we are dealing with the same basic needs; reduction of the active ingredient and the excipients so as to prevent cross-contamination and reduce the bioburden levels (for the next product or "run"). Cleaning is considered so important that the FDA has issued a guidance document just for this purpose.[7] This FDA guideline on Cleaning Validations outlines the approach the industry should be taking in order to complete this aspect of the program effectively.

Before any cleaning is performed thought must be given to the limits of the cleaning process. That is, "How clean is clean?" These limits are set based on the type of product and the means of application to the patient (solid oral dose, skin cream, parenteral). There is also a safety factor that needs to be considered. This safety factor is also based on the product type and the means of delivery. Parenterals often have a safety factor of 1000 (or greater) while skin creams that are not absorbed may have a safety factor around 10. Using these factors and other information one can calculate the amount of maximum carryover that would be allowed. The formula for this is:

$$MAC(O) = TDDp \times MBS/SF \times TDDn$$

TDDp (previous) = Standard therapeutic dose of the product (in the same dosage form as TDDnext
TDDn (next) = Standard therapeutic dose of the daily dose for the next product
MBS = Minimum batch size for the next product(s) (where MACO can end up)
SF Safety factor (eg, Topicals = 10, Solid Oral Dose = 100, Parenteral's = 1000 or higher)

GENERAL CLEANING CONSIDERATIONS

As with any validation program a cleaning validation master plan should be prepared in advance. In this document the manufacturer

Table 11.2 Determining the "Worst Case"					
Solubility	Toxicity	Dose	Interactions	Hardest to Clean	Microbiology
Water	Safety factor	Therapeutic	Next compound	Equipment	Storage
Solvents	Degradation products	Maximum	Process equipment	Product	
Detergent	Impurities		Excipients		
Other			API		

should describe the methods to be used for cleaning each piece of equipment. The plan should also give the frequency of cleaning and a plan for determining both clean and dirty hold times (clean hold—time after cleaning; dirty hold—time after use).

Also the level of carryover allowed based on the next product to be made in that equipment should be specified. If the manufacturer is not sure what the next product will be, that is, the company is a contract manufacturer, then the worst-case carryover should be used (ie, the lowest amount based on all possible products). The "worst-case" situation should always be used in determining the best cleaning procedure. Table 11.2 shows some of the considerations to be used in determining the worst-case for cleaning. For example, if a piece of equipment is very hard to clean and a procedure for its cleaning is established then that procedure can be used for all other pieces of equipment with the knowledge that they will also be cleaned.

Another approach to determine cleaning is to use a matrix format. This can be used when the products are similar in composition (all having the same ingredients but possible different concentrations of one or more). If this method is used, a scientific and statistical discussion should be made in the cleaning master plan.

FACILITY DESIGN AND CLEANING

When the facility is designed for pharmaceutical manufacturing several things need to be addressed. One is the size and layout (flow of materials and people), the second is its maintenance. Here, maintenance includes cleaning. 21 CFR 211.42(a) states that the building must be able to support proper operations that include cleaning.

Facility construction for the controlled areas includes cleanable walls, ceilings, and floors. Thus, smooth finishes are the standard in the industry. Another consideration in cleaning the facility is the flow of materials. This would include all materials coming in (raw materials), in-process materials moving through the facility, and waste material leaving the production areas (eg, component packaging). The use of closed transport containers will reduce the amount of dust and material during transport through the building.

To clean the facility one must consider the cleaning agents to be used. They must be effective in removing the materials that are volatile or due to dust dispersions from production. These "stick" to the room surfaces and need to be removed periodically in order to prevent cross-contamination. In addition, the bioburden tends to grow, especially if the relative humidity is over 50%. It is common practice to use three cleaning agents for the facility and to rotate them on a monthly basis. This prevents the bioburden from forming resistant strains. The effectiveness and completeness of this cleaning process also needs to be validated.

EQUIPMENT CLEANING

Certainly if the facility needs to be kept clean the process equipment needs attention.[8] There are two methods of cleaning the process equipment:

- Manual (best if the equipment needs to be disassembled)
- Automated or semiautomated (Clean in Place—CIP)

Manual cleaning is most likely the least expensive method, yet in the long term it may be the most expensive. There are some potential problems with the manual cleaning method:

- Can't reach all areas of the equipment—that is, large tanks
- Operator training is critical and can be highly variable
  - Even trained operators may vary their cleaning each time
- Possible risk to the operator by the cleaning agent(s) or the product residue

Using CIP for cleaning yields the most consistent results. However, as with the manual method there are some potential problems:

- Cost can be very high
- The equipment cannot be disassembled for cleaning
- Potential for contaminated cleaning fluids or rinse water to "re-dirty" the cleaned area

Regardless of the method chosen to clean the equipment, the cleaning process must be validated. The validation program for equipment cleaning is the same as all other validations. A protocol needs to be prepared with preplanned and quantifiable acceptance criteria. It must be reviewed and approved by the Quality unit prior to execution. The cleaning procedure should be developed and tested in the laboratory or pilot area prior to being used on the process equipment. Again, cleaning validation is not a development program. All testing and optimization (for both manual and CIP functions) need to be completed prior to the validation tests.

In addition to the validation of the cleaning procedures, the cleaning methods (analysis of the data) also need to be validated. Here, the methods used to determine "how clean" the unit is need to be validated just as the analytical methods need validation. In performing the validation[9] of the cleaning activity for Active Pharmaceutical Ingredients (APIs) or finished drug substances or products there are several considerations:

- Limit of Detection (LOD)
- Limit of Quantitation (LOQ)
- Specificity
  - Nonspecific—for example, Total Organic Carbon (TOC)
  - Specific—for example, Atomic Adsorption
- Robustness
- Operator to Operator consistency (Note: Less important if CIP is used)

OTHER CLEANING CONSIDERATIONS

As with process validation, cleaning validation needs samples in order to prove that the cleaning was and remains effective. The determination of the effectiveness, as stated, should have been done in the laboratory. The level at which the equipment is considered "clean" depends on several factors[10]:

- Toxicity
- Carryover to the next product (Need to calculate Maximum Carryover)
- Decomposition or metabolites formed during the process
- Mode of administration (Parenteral, Oral Solid Dose, etc.)
- State of the material (eg, solid, powder, liquid)

Another important consideration is the method of sampling. The FDA prefers direct sampling as this allows the detection of materials in hard to reach places and allows a direct correlation with the surface material (dirt). The drawback to the direct sampling method is that the swab used must be compatible with all of the product ingredients and the solvent used should not interfere with the analysis. In addition, a recovery test needs to be performed. The recovery test needs to be specific for the major or worst case "contaminant," usually the API. That is, the amount of material recovered from the swab (ie, after placing in the solvent tube) needs to be calculated. In general a 70% or better recovery is considered acceptable.

If the vessel is too large for direct sampling, or the system is a closed system (no access for swabbing) then a rinse sample is allowed. The rinse approach assumes that the material to be removed is fully soluble in the solvent used for the rinse. This needs to be demonstrated and documented in the laboratory. A quantitation of the rinse solution is then performed. It may be necessary to concentrate the rinse solution in order to obtain a valid reading of the concentration.

Also, if the rinse method of verifying the cleaning is used there needs to be a correlation between the swab and rinse approach. Taking a known quantity of the product and applying it to two coupons and allowing it to dry is used to accomplish this. One coupon is then rinsed with the same rinse solution, using the same flow rate and temperature as would be used on the equipment. The other coupon is swabbed and the material recovered from the swab tested and compared to the rinse sample.

NOTES

1. Title 21 Code of Federal Regulations Parts 210 and 211, 2015.

2. Classifications: 100,000 is 100,000 (etc.) particles of $<0.5 \, \mu/Ft^3$.

3. Depending on containment or other safety issues.

4. For products other than aseptic fills.

5. Note: Sanitary line should not be placed over process lines and joints in piping should be separated.

6. Ostrove, S.: Personal experience.

7. Guide to the Inspections Validation of Cleaning Processes; FDA Jul. 1993.

8. Haga, R., Murakami, S., Ostrove, S., Weiss, S.: Cleaning Mechanism Study for Bio-Pharmaceutical Plant Design, Pharmaceutical Engineering, Sep./Oct. 8−21, 1997.

9. Walsh, A.: Cleaning Validation for the 21st Century: Acceptance Limits for Active Pharmaceutical Ingredients (APIs) Part 1, Pharm Eng. Jul./Aug. 74−83, 2011 and Part II, Pharm. Eng. Sep./Oct. 46-49, 2011.

10. Bhattacharya, J.: Cleaning Validation Procedure and Limit Computation in Pharmaceutical Industry: An Ample Approach, Sep. 18, 2015, www.LinkedIn.com

The following commonly used terms are identified and defined:

Acceptance Criteria   A set of measurable qualities or specifications used to check out system or equipment installation, operation, or performance. Conformance with these qualities or specifications provides a high degree of confidence that a system is installed, operates, or performs as intended.

Accuracy   Expresses the closeness of agreement between the value that is accepted either as a conventional true value or an accepted reference value and the value found.

Air Lock   Two airtight doors with space inbetween them.

Alarm   Device or function that signals the existence of an abnormal condition by means of an audible or visual change or both.

ANSI   American National Standards Institute.

Approval (Approved)   A document has been approved after it has been reviewed and signed by a group of individuals representing the QA/QC, manufacturing, and engineering disciplines. Other disciplines may partake in the reviews as required.

API   Active Pharmaceutical Ingredient.

ASTM   American Society for Testing and Materials.

Audit or Quality Audit   A documented activity performed on a periodic basis in accordance with written procedures to verify, by examination and evaluation of the objective evidence, compliance with those elements of the quality program under review.

Calibration   Comparison of a measurement standard or instrument of known accuracy with another standard or instrument to detect, correlate, report, and/or eliminate any variation in the accuracy of the item being compared.

CDER   Center for Drug Evaluation and Research.

Certification   Documented testimony by qualified personnel that a system qualification, validation or revalidation has been performed appropriately and that the results are acceptable.

CFR   Code of Federal Regulations.

CGMP (GMP)   Current Good Manufacturing Practice.

Change Control   A formalized program by which qualified representatives review proposed and actual changes to products, processes, equipment, or software to determine their potential impact on the validation status. It provides an audit trail of changes made.

Characteristic   A physical, chemical, functional identifiable property of the product, component, or raw material.

Clean-In-Place (CIP)   A system of pumps, tanks, and distribution piping designed to circulate detergents, disinfectants, and flushing liquids through process equipment systems without disassembling, hand-cleaning, and reassembling the system. CIP systems can be semiautomatically or fully automatically controlled.

Compendial Test Methods   Test methods that appear in official compendia such as the United States Pharmacopoeia (USP).

Component   Any material, substance, part, or assembly used during product manufacture that is intended to be included in the finished product.

Concurrent Validation   The validation process whereby the equipment or process is tested and qualified during actual production or regular use.

Controls Testing   Testing that verifies switches, controls, and soft keys located on the control panel or associated with FCS operate as designed and in conjunction with equipment and operating parameters.

Control Parameter Those operating variables that are utilized to specify conditions under which the product is to be manufactured.

Critical Instrumentation Any instrument that provides a record of the process that is used in determining quality of the product.

Critical Process Parameter (CPP) A process parameter that must be met in order to meet the expectations of the process so that the product meets its intended criteria (CQA). A change in a CPP results in a change in a CQA.

Critical Quality Attribute (CQA) A measurable condition that must be met to assure product integrity in structure and or function. It may be an intermediate stage in the product production and be required to reach the next step or stage.

Critical System A system whose performance has a direct and measurable impact on the quality of the product. A system determined to be a critical system must be designated as such and operated and maintained per approved procedures.

Design Review A planned, scheduled, and documented audit of pertinent design aspects that can affect performance, safety or effectiveness.

Detection Limit The lowest amount of analyte in a sample that can be detected but not necessarily quantitated as an exact value.

Environment The condition, circumstances, influences, and stresses surrounding and affecting the product during storage, handling, transportation, installation, and use.

FAT Factory Acceptance Testing.

FDA Food and Drug Administration.

Functional Testing Testing that includes manual and automatic testing verifying components within the system (valves, etc.) and the system as a whole operates as designed and in conjunction with equipment and operating parameters.

FRS Functional Requirements Specifications.

Hardware	The physical components of an electronic control system (as contrasted with the software components). These components provide the physical connections to the system(s) or equipment to be controlled. Hardware components include (but are not limited to) the CPU (central processing unit—microprocessor), I/O (input/output—sensors, printers) and relays.
HEPA Filters	High Efficiency Particulate Air Filters.
HPLC	High performance liquid chromatography, or, High pressure liquid chromatography.
HVAC	Heating, ventilation and air conditioning.
ICH	International Council on Harmonization.
Installation Qualification (IQ)	Documented verification that key aspects of the installation adhere to appropriate codes, approved design specifications, and manufacturer's recommendations (where appropriate).
LAL	Limulous Amobysite Assay. The test used to determine endotoxin levels in a sample.
Laboratory Qualification	The process by which the staff, instrumentation, and all relevant support systems in a laboratory are demonstrated to be capable of carrying out a test method and consistently generate correct results in accordance with predetermined acceptance criteria.
Ladder Logic	A diagrammatically representation of the specific functions of an electronic control system for PLCs.
Linearity	Is the assay's ability (within a given range) to obtain test results that are directly proportional to the concentration (amount) of analyte in the sample.
Method Development	The process by which new methods are developed and evaluated for suitability of use as test methods.
Method Transfer	The process by which methods are transferred from the transferring laboratory to receiving laboratories such that performance

characteristics are retained within defined acceptance criteria. The transfer process should include qualification of the laboratory to use the method.

Method Validation
The process by which attributes such as accuracy, precision, selectivity, ruggedness, and reproducibility of developed methods are formally established against predefined acceptance criteria and documented. Except for stability indication, compendial methods may only require abbreviated method validation studies (eg, accuracy, linearity, bias, etc.).

NIST
National Institute of Standards and Technology.

"Noncritical" Instrumentation
Instrumentation used primarily for convenience, operator ease, or maintenance.

Operating Parameter or Variable
Those process variables which are measured to monitor the state of the process.

Operational Qualification (OQ)
Documented verification that systems or subsystems, capable of being changed, perform as intended throughout anticipated operating ranges.

OSHA
Occupational Safety and Health Administration.

P&ID
Piping and Instrumentation Drawing (Schematic representation of the installed piping and instruments).

Performance Qualification (PQ)
Documented verification that equipment, systems, or processes perform as intended throughout specified operating ranges.

pH
Logarithmic measurement of the acidity or alkalinity of a solution.

PLC
Programmed Logic Controller.

Precision
Expresses the closeness of agreement (degree of scatter) between a series of measurements obtained from sampling of the same homogenous sample under the prescribed conditions. Precision may be considered at three levels: repeatability, intermediate precision, and reproducibility.

Protocol	Written testing plan that includes the objectives and methods for the conduct of a study.
PPQ	Process Performance Qualification.
Process Validation (now Process Performance Qualification PPQ)	Obtaining documented evidence that the process or production of the pharmaceutical product meets the pre-approved acceptance criteria for that product.
Prospective Validation (Validation)	A defined strategy of test procedures which in combination with routine production methods and quality control techniques provides documented assurance that a system is performing as intended and/or that a product conforms to its predetermined specifications.
Preventative Maintenance	The program or procedures used to keep all process systems fully operating within accepted predefined specifications.
Proven Acceptable Range (PAR)	Those values of a control or operating parameter that fall between the proven upper and lower operating conditions (validated ranges). The PAR values are derived from developmental validation studies whose intent is, primarily, to establish the operational ranges to be used in the production environment.
Software	The portion of an electronic control system comprised of instructions written in one or more artificial language(s). Some are readable as standard English and others, binary for example, that are only readable by machine or those extremely well versed in the "machine language." These instructions provide the specific directions to the electronic control system to perform various functions. Software is frequently user (or self) alterable. This alterability of software results in greater flexibility of the system and greater risk. This risk is offset by instigating software change control measures, security access, and using compiled code.

Source Code The code used by computers or controllers of process systems or equipment. This code is readable only by the machine components themselves (frequently this code is binary) and can be very specific to the particular machine components in question. Most humans cannot write software directly in machine-readable (compiled) code, therefore, humans typically write code in a higher order language such as Cobol, Fortran, etc. This human readable code is called the source code (because it is the source of the machine-readable code). This source code is compiled (translated) by a computer system from the human readable form to the machine-readable form.

Startup/ Commissioning (S/C) The program or procedure used to perform preliminary testing on equipment or utilities. It provides documentation that the equipment is connected according to design specifications; and that the basic operation is achievable.

Standard Operating Procedure (SOP) Written instructions that enable a trained person to operate or otherwise perform a given function.

Qualification The procedure by which equipment, processes and instrumentation are proven to be designed properly and perform adequately and reproducibility as designed.

Quality The composite of the characteristics, including performance, of an item or product.

Quality Assurance (QA) Program Requirements As defined in the GMP, the requirements consist of procedures adequate to assure the quality of the manufacturing process and adequate to assure that the following functions are performed: (1) review of production records; (2) approval or rejection of components, drug product containers, closures, in-process materials, packaging materials, labeling, and drug products: approval or rejection of drug products manufactured, processed, packaged, or held under contract by another company;

(3) availability of adequate laboratory facilities for testing and, based on test results, determining disposition of components, drug product containers, closures, packaging materials, in-process materials, and drug products; and (4) approval or rejection of procedures and specifications impacting on the strength, quality, and purity of the drug product.

Quality Control (QC) Unit
A regulatory process whereby the quality of raw materials and produced product is controlled by inspection and tested for the purpose of preventing production of defective product. This unit is comprised of QA and QC.

Qualification of Methods
The process by which methods are determined to be suitable for analysis of a given test article by a given laboratory.

Quantitation limit
Is the lowest amount of analyte in a sample that can be quantitatively determined with suitable precision and accuracy.

Quarantine
Any area that is marked, designated, or set aside for the holding of incoming components prior to acceptance examination and finished products until released.

Range
is the interval between the upper and lower concentration (amounts) of analyte in the sample (including these concentrations) for which it has been demonstrated that the analytical procedure has a suitable level of precision, accuracy, and linearity.

Reference Instrumentation
Any instrument excluded from the calibration program because of its inability to be calibrated or its infrequency of use.

Regulatory Test Method
A test method that has been approved by a governmental regulatory agency such as the FDA.

Repeatability
Expresses the precision under the same operating conditions over a short interval of time. Repeatability is also referred to as "intra-assay precision."

Reproducibility Expresses the precision between laboratories (collaborative studies, usually applied to standardization of methodology).

Retrospective Validation Performing analysis on previous batch records for a given operation. A sufficient number of batches or production runs must be used in the analysis in order to demonstrate reproducibility and compliance with CGMP regulations overall.

Rework A set of procedures that define the conditions under which a process or batch of product can be mixed into or otherwise redone so as to make it conform to the required specifications for that product.

Robustness Is a measure of the assay's capacity to remain unaffected by small but deliberate variations in method parameters and provides an indication of its reliability during normal usage.

R&D Research and Development.

Revalidation The repetition of the validation process or a specific portion of it, to assure that a system is suitable for use after modification or repair. Revalidation is required on a periodic basis to ensure that the process or system continues to operate as intended.

Sanitization Reduction in the number of microorganisms to a safe or relatively safe level as determined by applicable regulations or the purpose of application.

Sanitizer Any chemical that kills microbial contamination in the form of vegetative cells.

Specificity Is the ability to assess unequivocally the analyte in the presence of components that may be expected to be present. Typically these might include impurities, degradants, matrices, etc.

State of Control A condition in which operating and control parameters of processes or systems are stable and within ranges documented to establish consistent and reliable control of the processes.

System	A number of integrated steps, functions, and items of equipment that must be considered as a unit in order to assure supply of a consistent, uniform, and high quality component for the manufacture of a product.
System Suitability	Specific tests designed to determine the suitability of the overall test system (including instrumentation, sample preparation, and analyst) is suitable for the intended use of the test method. Typical tests utilized for system suitability measure test system precision, specificity, and detection.
Transfer Area	Any area of the manufacturing facility, other than the weighing, mixing, or filling areas, where the components, in-process materials, and drug products, and drug product contact surfaces of equipment, containers, and closures after final rinse of such surfaces, are exposed to the plant environment.
Testing	Qualified activities performed by the testing laboratory, utilizing approved, validated, qualified, and (if appropriate) successfully transferred methods. These activities accomplish the purpose of establishing testing procedures to ensure accurate determination of the identity, strength, quality, and purity of the component/product tested.
Testing Laboratory	The laboratory that performs routine testing for official disposition (eg, release, stability) of components and/or products. The testing laboratory may be a QA laboratory at a manufacturing site or a contract laboratory whose use is approved in accord with corporate policies/procedures.
Test Method	An approved detailed procedure describing how to test a sample for a specified attribute (eg, assay), the amount required, instrumentation, reagents, sample preparation steps, data generation steps, and calculations used for evaluation.

Test Results	The final calculated results obtained after testing has been completed.
USP	United States Pharmacopoeia.
Validation Change Control	A formalized program by which qualified representatives review proposed and actual changes to products, processes, equipment, and/or software to determine their potential impact on the validation status. Based on impact determinations action is taken that ensures the system retains its validated state.
Validation Protocol	An approved document stating how validation is conducted. The document includes test parameters, product characteristics, required equipment and procedures, and acceptance criteria.
Validation Final Report	An approved document of the results derived from executing a validation protocol. The report includes a brief summary of conclusions based on test results of the validation status. Proven acceptable ranges for critical process parameters are designated as determined by the results of the validation study.
Verify	Comparison of a measurement standard of known accuracy with another standard or instrument to detect, correlate, or report, but not eliminate, any variation in the accuracy of the item being compared. Verification implies that no adjustment of the compared item is possible to reestablish accuracy.
"Worst Case"	A set of conditions encompassing upper and lower processing limits and circumstances, including those within standard operating procedures, which pose the greatest chance of process or product failure when compared to ideal conditions. Such conditions do not necessarily induce product or process failure.

APPENDIX *A*

21 CFR 211

Code of Federal Regulations
[Title 21, Volume 4]
[Revised as of April 1, 2015]
[CITE: 21CFR211]

TITLE 21--FOOD AND DRUGS
CHAPTER I--FOOD AND DRUG ADMINISTRATION
DEPARTMENT OF HEALTH AND HUMAN SERVICES
SUBCHAPTER C--DRUGS: GENERAL

PART 211 CURRENT GOOD MANUFACTURING PRACTICE
FOR FINISHED PHARMACEUTICALS

Subpart A--General Provisions

Sec. 211.1 Scope.

(a) The regulations in this part contain the minimum current good manufacturing practice for preparation of drug products (excluding positron emission tomography drugs) for administration to humans or animals.

(b) The current good manufacturing practice regulations in this chapter as they pertain to drug products; in parts 600 through 680 of this chapter, as they pertain to drugs that are also biological products for human use; and in part 1271 of this chapter, as they are applicable to drugs that are also human cells, tissues, and cellular and tissue-based products (HCT/Ps) and that are drugs (subject to review under an application submitted under section 505 of the act or under a biological product license application under section 351 of the Public Health Service Act); supplement and do not supersede the regulations in this part unless the regulations explicitly provide otherwise. In the event of a conflict between applicable regulations in this part and in other parts of this chapter, or in parts 600 through 680 of this chapter, or in part 1271 of this chapter, the regulation specifically applicable to the drug product in question shall supersede the more general.

(c) Pending consideration of a proposed exemption, published in the Federal Register of September 29, 1978, the requirements in this part shall not be enforced for OTC drug products if the products and all their ingredients are ordinarily marketed and consumed as human foods, and which products may also fall within the legal definition of drugs by virtue of their intended use. Therefore, until further notice, regulations under part 110 of this chapter, and where applicable, parts 113 to 129 of this chapter, shall be applied in determining whether these OTC drug products that are also foods are manufactured, processed, packed, or held under current good manufacturing practice.

Sec. 211.3 Definitions.

The definitions set forth in 210.3 of this chapter apply in this part.

Subpart B--Organization and Personnel

Sec. 211.22 Responsibilities of quality control unit.

(a) There shall be a quality control unit that shall have the responsibility and authority to approve or reject all components, drug product containers, closures, in-process materials, packaging material, labeling, and drug products, and the authority to review production records to assure that no errors have occurred or, if errors have occurred, that they have been fully investigated. The quality control unit shall be responsible for approving or rejecting drug products manufactured, processed, packed, or held under contract by another company.

(b) Adequate laboratory facilities for the testing and approval (or rejection) of components, drug product containers, closures, packaging materials, in-process materials, and drug products shall be available to the quality control unit.

(c) The quality control unit shall have the responsibility for approving or rejecting all procedures or specifications impacting on the identity, strength, quality, and purity of the drug product.

(d) The responsibilities and procedures applicable to the quality control unit shall be in writing; such written procedures shall be followed.

Sec. 211.25 Personnel qualifications.

(a) Each person engaged in the manufacture, processing, packing, or holding of a drug product shall have education, training, and experience, or any combination thereof, to enable that person to perform the assigned functions. Training shall be in the particular operations that the employee performs and in current good manufacturing practice (including the current good manufacturing practice regulations in this chapter and written procedures required by these regulations) as they relate to the employee's functions. Training in current good manufacturing practice shall be conducted by qualified individuals on a continuing basis and with sufficient frequency to assure that employees remain familiar with CGMP requirements applicable to them.

(b) Each person responsible for supervising the manufacture, processing, packing, or holding of a drug product shall have the education, training, and experience, or any combination thereof, to perform assigned functions in such a manner as to provide assurance that the drug product has the safety, identity, strength, quality, and purity that it purports or is represented to possess.

(c) There shall be an adequate number of qualified personnel to perform and supervise the manufacture, processing, packing, or holding of each drug product.

Sec. 211.28 Personnel responsibilities.

(a) Personnel engaged in the manufacture, processing, packing, or holding of a drug product shall wear clean clothing appropriate for the duties they perform. Protective apparel, such as head, face, hand, and arm coverings, shall be worn as necessary to protect drug products from contamination.

(b) Personnel shall practice good sanitation and health habits.

(c) Only personnel authorized by supervisory personnel shall enter those areas of the buildings and facilities designated as limited-access areas.

(d) Any person shown at any time (either by medical examination or supervisory observation) to have an apparent illness or open lesions that may adversely affect the safety or quality of drug products shall be excluded from direct contact with components, drug product containers, closures, in-process materials, and drug products until the condition is corrected or determined by competent medical personnel not to jeopardize the safety or quality of drug products. All personnel shall be instructed to report to supervisory personnel any health conditions that may have an adverse effect on drug products.

Sec. 211.34 Consultants.

Consultants advising on the manufacture, processing, packing, or holding of drug products shall have sufficient education, training, and experience, or any combination thereof, to advise on the subject for which they are retained. Records shall be maintained stating the name, address, and qualifications of any consultants and the type of service they provide.

Subpart C--Buildings and Facilities

Sec. 211.42 Design and construction features.

(a) Any building or buildings used in the manufacture, processing, packing, or holding of a drug product shall be of suitable size, construction and location to facilitate cleaning, maintenance, and proper operations.

(b) Any such building shall have adequate space for the orderly placement of equipment and materials to prevent mixups between different components, drug product containers, closures, labeling, in-process materials, or drug products, and to prevent contamination. The flow of components, drug product containers, closures, labeling, in-process materials, and drug products through the building or buildings shall be designed to prevent contamination.

(c) Operations shall be performed within specifically defined areas of adequate size. There shall be separate or defined areas or such other control systems for the firm's operations as are necessary to prevent contamination or mixups during the course of the following procedures:

(1) Receipt, identification, storage, and withholding from use of components, drug product containers, closures, and labeling, pending the appropriate sampling, testing, or examination by the quality control unit before release for manufacturing or packaging;

(2) Holding rejected components, drug product containers, closures, and labeling before disposition;

(3) Storage of released components, drug product containers, closures, and labeling;

(4) Storage of in-process materials;

(5) Manufacturing and processing operations;

(6) Packaging and labeling operations;

(7) Quarantine storage before release of drug products;

(8) Storage of drug products after release;

(9) Control and laboratory operations;

(10) Aseptic processing, which includes as appropriate:

(i) Floors, walls, and ceilings of smooth, hard surfaces that are easily cleanable;

(ii) Temperature and humidity controls;

(iii) An air supply filtered through high-efficiency particulate air filters under positive pressure, regardless of whether flow is laminar or nonlaminar;

(iv) A system for monitoring environmental conditions;

(v) A system for cleaning and disinfecting the room and equipment to produce aseptic conditions;

(vi) A system for maintaining any equipment used to control the aseptic conditions.

(d) Operations relating to the manufacture, processing, and packing of penicillin shall be performed in facilities separate from those used for other drug products for human use.

Sec. 211.44 Lighting.

Adequate lighting shall be provided in all areas.

Sec. 211.46 Ventilation, air filtration, air heating and cooling.

(a) Adequate ventilation shall be provided.

(b) Equipment for adequate control over air pressure, microorganisms, dust, humidity, and temperature shall be provided when appropriate for the manufacture, processing, packing, or holding of a drug product.

(c) Air filtration systems, including prefilters and particulate matter air filters, shall be used when appropriate on air supplies to production areas. If air is recirculated to production areas, measures shall be taken to control recirculation of dust from production. In areas where air contamination occurs during production, there shall be adequate exhaust systems or other systems adequate to control contaminants.

(d) Air-handling systems for the manufacture, processing, and packing of penicillin shall be completely separate from those for other drug products for human use.

Sec. 211.48 Plumbing.

(a) Potable water shall be supplied under continuous positive pressure in a plumbing system free of defects that could contribute contamination to any drug product. Potable water shall meet the standards prescribed in the Environmental Protection Agency's Primary Drinking Water Regulations set forth in 40 CFR part 141. Water not meeting such standards shall not be permitted in the potable water system.

(b) Drains shall be of adequate size and, where connected directly to a sewer, shall be provided with an air break or other mechanical device to prevent back-siphonage.

Sec. 211.50 Sewage and refuse.

Sewage, trash, and other refuse in and from the building and immediate premises shall be disposed of in a safe and sanitary manner.

Sec. 211.52 Washing and toilet facilities.

Adequate washing facilities shall be provided, including hot and cold water, soap or detergent, air driers or single-service towels, and clean toilet facilities easily accesible to working areas.

Sec. 211.56 Sanitation.

(a) Any building used in the manufacture, processing, packing, or holding of a drug product shall be maintained in a clean and sanitary condition, Any such building shall be free of infestation by rodents, birds, insects, and other vermin (other than laboratory animals). Trash and organic waste matter shall be held and disposed of in a timely and sanitary manner.

(b) There shall be written procedures assigning responsibility for sanitation and describing in sufficient detail the cleaning schedules, methods, equipment, and materials to be used in cleaning the buildings and facilities; such written procedures shall be followed.

(c) There shall be written procedures for use of suitable rodenticides, insecticides, fungicides, fumigating agents, and cleaning and sanitizing agents. Such written procedures shall be designed to prevent the contamination of equipment, components, drug product containers, closures, packaging, labeling materials, or drug products and shall be followed. Rodenticides, insecticides, and fungicides shall not be used unless registered and used in accordance with the Federal Insecticide, Fungicide, and Rodenticide Act (7 U.S.C. 135).

(d) Sanitation procedures shall apply to work performed by contractors or temporary employees as well as work performed by full-time employees during the ordinary course of operations.

Sec. 211.58 Maintenance.

Any building used in the manufacture, processing, packing, or holding of a drug product shall be maintained in a good state of repair.

Subpart D--Equipment

Sec. 211.63 Equipment design, size, and location.

Equipment used in the manufacture, processing, packing, or holding of a drug product shall be of appropriate design, adequate size, and suitably located to facilitate operations for its intended use and for its cleaning and maintenance.

Sec. 211.65 Equipment construction.

(a) Equipment shall be constructed so that surfaces that contact components, in-process materials, or drug products shall not be reactive, additive, or absorptive so as to alter the safety, identity, strength, quality, or purity of the drug product beyond the official or other established requirements.

(b) Any substances required for operation, such as lubricants or coolants, shall not come into contact with components, drug product containers, closures, in-process materials, or drug products so as to alter the safety, identity, strength, quality, or purity of the drug product beyond the official or other established requirements.

Sec. 211.67 Equipment cleaning and maintenance.

(a) Equipment and utensils shall be cleaned, maintained, and, as appropriate for the nature of the drug, sanitized and/or sterilized at appropriate intervals to prevent malfunctions or contamination that would alter the safety, identity, strength, quality, or purity of the drug product beyond the official or other established requirements.

(b) Written procedures shall be established and followed for cleaning and maintenance of equipment, including utensils, used in the manufacture, processing, packing, or holding of a drug product. These procedures shall include, but are not necessarily limited to, the following:

(1) Assignment of responsibility for cleaning and maintaining equipment;

(2) Maintenance and cleaning schedules, including, where appropriate, sanitizing schedules;

(3) A description in sufficient detail of the methods, equipment, and materials used in cleaning and maintenance operations, and the methods of disassembling and reassembling equipment as necessary to assure proper cleaning and maintenance;

(4) Removal or obliteration of previous batch identification;

(5) Protection of clean equipment from contamination prior to use;

(6) Inspection of equipment for cleanliness immediately before use.

(c) Records shall be kept of maintenance, cleaning, sanitizing, and inspection as specified in 211.180 and 211.182.

Sec. 211.68 Automatic, mechanical, and electronic equipment.

(a) Automatic, mechanical, or electronic equipment or other types of equipment, including computers, or related systems that will perform a function satisfactorily, may be used in the manufacture, processing, packing, and holding of a drug product. If such equipment is so used, it shall be routinely calibrated, inspected, or checked according to a written program designed to assure proper performance. Written records of those calibration checks and inspections shall be maintained.

(b) Appropriate controls shall be exercised over computer or related systems to assure that changes in master production and control records or other records are instituted only by authorized personnel. Input to and output from the computer or related system of formulas or other records or data shall be checked for accuracy. The degree and frequency of input/output verification shall be based on the complexity and reliability of the computer or related system. A backup file of data entered into the computer or related system shall be maintained except where certain data, such as calculations performed in connection with laboratory analysis, are eliminated by computerization or other automated processes. In such instances a written record of the program shall be maintained along with appropriate validation data. Hard copy or alternative systems, such as duplicates, tapes, or microfilm, designed to assure that backup data are exact and complete and that it is secure from alteration, inadvertent erasures, or loss shall be maintained.

(c) Such automated equipment used for performance of operations addressed by 211.101(c) or (d), 211.103, 211.182, or 211.188(b)(11) can satisfy the requirements included in those sections relating to the performance of an operation by one person and checking by another person if such equipment is used in conformity with this section, and one person checks that the equipment properly performed the operation.

Sec. 211.72 Filters.

Filters for liquid filtration used in the manufacture, processing, or packing of injectable drug products intended for human use shall not release fibers into such products. Fiber-releasing filters may be used when it is not possible to manufacture such products without the use of these filters. If use of a fiber-releasing filter is necessary, an additional nonfiber-releasing filter having a maximum nominal pore size rating of 0.2 micron (0.45 micron if the manufacturing conditions so dictate) shall subsequently be used to reduce the content of particles in the injectable drug product. The use of an asbestos-containing filter is prohibited.

Subpart E--Control of Components and Drug Product Containers and Closures

Sec. 211.80 General requirements.

(a) There shall be written procedures describing in sufficient detail the receipt, identification, storage, handling, sampling, testing, and approval or rejection of components and drug product containers and closures; such written procedures shall be followed.

(b) Components and drug product containers and closures shall at all times be handled and stored in a manner to prevent contamination.

(c) Bagged or boxed components of drug product containers, or closures shall be stored off the floor and suitably spaced to permit cleaning and inspection.

(d) Each container or grouping of containers for components or drug product containers, or closures shall be identified with a distinctive code for each lot in each shipment received. This code shall be used in recording the disposition of each lot. Each lot shall be appropriately identified as to its status (i.e., quarantined, approved, or rejected).

Sec. 211.82 Receipt and storage of untested components, drug product containers, and closures.

(a) Upon receipt and before acceptance, each container or grouping of containers of components, drug product containers, and closures shall be examined visually for appropriate labeling as to contents, container damage or broken seals, and contamination.

(b) Components, drug product containers, and closures shall be stored under quarantine until they have been tested or examined, whichever is appropriate, and released. Storage within the area shall conform to the requirements of 211.80.

Sec. 211.84 Testing and approval or rejection of components, drug product containers, and closures.

(a) Each lot of components, drug product containers, and closures shall be withheld from use until the lot has been sampled, tested, or examined, as appropriate, and released for use by the quality control unit.

(b) Representative samples of each shipment of each lot shall be collected for testing or examination. The number of containers to be sampled, and the amount of material to be taken from each container, shall be based upon appropriate criteria such as statistical criteria for component variability, confidence levels, and degree of precision desired, the past quality history of the supplier, and the quantity needed for analysis and reserve where required by 211.170.

(c) Samples shall be collected in accordance with the following procedures:

(1) The containers of components selected shall be cleaned when necessary in a manner to prevent introduction of contaminants into the component.

(2) The containers shall be opened, sampled, and resealed in a manner designed to prevent contamination of their contents and contamination of other components, drug product containers, or closures.

(3) Sterile equipment and aseptic sampling techniques shall be used when necessary.

(4) If it is necessary to sample a component from the top, middle, and bottom of its container, such sample subdivisions shall not be composited for testing.

(5) Sample containers shall be identified so that the following information can be determined: name of the material sampled, the lot number, the container from which the sample was taken, the date on which the sample was taken, and the name of the person who collected the sample.

(6) Containers from which samples have been taken shall be marked to show that samples have been removed from them.

(d) Samples shall be examined and tested as follows:

(1) At least one test shall be conducted to verify the identity of each component of a drug product. Specific identity tests, if they exist, shall be used.

(2) Each component shall be tested for conformity with all appropriate written specifications for purity, strength, and quality. In lieu of

such testing by the manufacturer, a report of analysis may be accepted from the supplier of a component, provided that at least one specific identity test is conducted on such component by the manufacturer, and provided that the manufacturer establishes the reliability of the supplier's analyses through appropriate validation of the supplier's test results at appropriate intervals.

(3) Containers and closures shall be tested for conformity with all appropriate written specifications. In lieu of such testing by the manufacturer, a certificate of testing may be accepted from the supplier, provided that at least a visual identification is conducted on such containers/closures by the manufacturer and provided that the manufacturer establishes the reliability of the supplier's test results through appropriate validation of the supplier's test results at appropriate intervals.

(4) When appropriate, components shall be microscopically examined.

(5) Each lot of a component, drug product container, or closure that is liable to contamination with filth, insect infestation, or other extraneous adulterant shall be examined against established specifications for such contamination.

(6) Each lot of a component, drug product container, or closure with potential for microbiological contamination that is objectionable in view of its intended use shall be subjected to microbiological tests before use.

(e) Any lot of components, drug product containers, or closures that meets the appropriate written specifications of identity, strength, quality, and purity and related tests under paragraph (d) of this section may be approved and released for use. Any lot of such material that does not meet such specifications shall be rejected.

Sec. 211.86 Use of approved components, drug product containers, and closures.

Components, drug product containers, and closures approved for use shall be rotated so that the oldest approved stock is used first. Deviation from this requirement is permitted if such deviation is temporary and appropriate.

Sec. 211.87 Retesting of approved components, drug product containers, and closures.

Components, drug product containers, and closures shall be retested or reexamined, as appropriate, for identity, strength, quality, and purity and approved or rejected by the quality control unit in accordance with 211.84 as necessary, e.g., after storage for long periods or after exposure to air, heat or other conditions that might adversely affect the component, drug product container, or closure.

Sec. 211.89 Rejected components, drug product containers, and closures.

Rejected components, drug product containers, and closures shall be identified and controlled under a quarantine system designed to prevent their use in manufacturing or processing operations for which they are unsuitable.

Sec. 211.94 Drug product containers and closures.

(a) Drug product containers and closures shall not be reactive, additive, or absorptive so as to alter the safety, identity, strength, quality, or purity of the drug beyond the official or established requirements.

(b) Container closure systems shall provide adequate protection against foreseeable external factors in storage and use that can cause deterioration or contamination of the drug product.

(c) Drug product containers and closures shall be clean and, where indicated by the nature of the drug, sterilized and processed to remove pyrogenic properties to assure that they are suitable for their intended use. Such depyrogenation processes shall be validated.

(d) Standards or specifications, methods of testing, and, where indicated, methods of cleaning, sterilizing, and processing to remove pyrogenic properties shall be written and followed for drug product containers and closures.

Subpart F--Production and Process Controls

Sec. 211.100 Written procedures; deviations.

(a) There shall be written procedures for production and process control designed to assure that the drug products have the identity, strength, quality, and purity they purport or are represented to possess. Such procedures shall include all requirements in this subpart. These written procedures, including any changes, shall be drafted, reviewed, and approved by the appropriate organizational units and reviewed and approved by the quality control unit.

(b) Written production and process control procedures shall be followed in the execution of the various production and process control functions and shall be documented at the time of performance. Any deviation from the written procedures shall be recorded and justified.

Sec. 211.101 Charge-in of components.

Written production and control procedures shall include the following, which are designed to assure that the drug products produced have the identity, strength, quality, and purity they purport or are represented to possess:

(a) The batch shall be formulated with the intent to provide not less than 100 percent of the labeled or established amount of active ingredient.

(b) Components for drug product manufacturing shall be weighed, measured, or subdivided as appropriate. If a component is removed from the original container to another, the new container shall be identified with the following information:

(1) Component name or item code;

(2) Receiving or control number;

(3) Weight or measure in new container;

(4) Batch for which component was dispensed, including its product name, strength, and lot number.

(c) Weighing, measuring, or subdividing operations for components shall be adequately supervised. Each container of component dispensed to manufacturing shall be examined by a second person to assure that:

(1) The component was released by the quality control unit;

(2) The weight or measure is correct as stated in the batch production records;

(3) The containers are properly identified. If the weighing, measuring, or subdividing operations are performed by automated equipment under 211.68, only one person is needed to assure paragraphs (c)(1), (c)(2), and (c)(3) of this section.

(d) Each component shall either be added to the batch by one person and verified by a second person or, if the components are added by automated equipment under 211.68, only verified by one person.

Sec. 211.103 Calculation of yield.

Actual yields and percentages of theoretical yield shall be determined at the conclusion of each appropriate phase of manufacturing, processing, packaging, or holding of the drug product. Such calculations shall either be performed by one person and independently verified by a second person, or, if the yield is calculated by automated equipment under 211.68, be independently verified by one person.

Sec. 211.105 Equipment identification.

(a) All compounding and storage containers, processing lines, and major equipment used during the production of a batch of a drug product shall be properly identified at all times to indicate their contents and, when necessary, the phase of processing of the batch.

(b) Major equipment shall be identified by a distinctive identification number or code that shall be recorded in the batch production record to show the specific equipment used in the manufacture of each batch of a drug product. In cases where only one of a particular type of equipment exists in a manufacturing facility, the name of the equipment may be used in lieu of a distinctive identification number or code.

Sec. 211.110 Sampling and testing of in-process materials and drug products.

(a) To assure batch uniformity and integrity of drug products, written procedures shall be established and followed that describe the in-process controls, and tests, or examinations to be conducted on appropriate samples of in-process materials of each batch. Such control procedures shall be established to monitor the output and to validate the performance of those manufacturing processes that may be responsible for causing variability in the characteristics of in-process material and the drug product. Such control procedures shall include, but are not limited to, the following, where appropriate:

(1) Tablet or capsule weight variation;

(2) Disintegration time;

(3) Adequacy of mixing to assure uniformity and homogeneity;

(4) Dissolution time and rate;

(5) Clarity, completeness, or pH of solutions.

(6) Bioburden testing.

(b) Valid in-process specifications for such characteristics shall be consistent with drug product final specifications and shall be derived from previous acceptable process average and process variability estimates where possible and determined by the application of suitable statistical procedures where appropriate. Examination and testing of samples shall assure that the drug product and in-process material conform to specifications.

(c) In-process materials shall be tested for identity, strength, quality, and purity as appropriate, and approved or rejected by the quality control unit, during the production process, e.g., at commencement or completion of significant phases or after storage for long periods.

(d) Rejected in-process materials shall be identified and controlled under a quarantine system designed to prevent their use in manufacturing or processing operations for which they are unsuitable.

Sec. 211.111 Time limitations on production.

When appropriate, time limits for the completion of each phase of production shall be established to assure the quality of the drug product. Deviation from established time limits may be acceptable if such deviation does not compromise the quality of the drug product. Such deviation shall be justified and documented.

Sec. 211.113 Control of microbiological contamination.

(a) Appropriate written procedures, designed to prevent objectionable microorganisms in drug products not required to be sterile, shall be established and followed.

(b) Appropriate written procedures, designed to prevent microbiological contamination of drug products purporting to be sterile, shall be established and followed. Such procedures shall include validation of all aseptic and sterilization processes.

Sec. 211.115 Reprocessing.

(a) Written procedures shall be established and followed prescribing a system for reprocessing batches that do not conform to standards or specifications and the steps to be taken to insure that the reprocessed batches will conform with all established standards, specifications, and characteristics.

(b) Reprocessing shall not be performed without the review and approval of the quality control unit.

Subpart G--Packaging and Labeling Control

Sec. 211.122 Materials examination and usage criteria.

(a) There shall be written procedures describing in sufficient detail the receipt, identification, storage, handling, sampling, examination, and/or testing of labeling and packaging materials; such written procedures shall be followed. Labeling and packaging materials shall be representatively sampled, and examined or tested upon receipt and before use in packaging or labeling of a drug product.

(b) Any labeling or packaging materials meeting appropriate written specifications may be approved and released for use. Any labeling or packaging materials that do not meet such specifications shall be rejected to prevent their use in operations for which they are unsuitable.

(c) Records shall be maintained for each shipment received of each different labeling and packaging material indicating receipt, examination or testing, and whether accepted or rejected.

(d) Labels and other labeling materials for each different drug product, strength, dosage form, or quantity of contents shall be stored separately with suitable identification. Access to the storage area shall be limited to authorized personnel.

(e) Obsolete and outdated labels, labeling, and other packaging materials shall be destroyed.

(f) Use of gang-printed labeling for different drug products, or different strengths or net contents of the same drug product, is prohibited unless the labeling from gang-printed sheets is adequately differentiated by size, shape, or color.

(g) If cut labeling is used for immediate container labels, individual unit cartons, or multiunit cartons containing immediate containers that are not packaged in individual unit cartons, packaging and labeling operations shall include one of the following special control procedures:

(1) Dedication of labeling and packaging lines to each different strength of each different drug product;

(2) Use of appropriate electronic or electromechanical equipment to conduct a 100-percent examination for correct labeling during or after completion of finishing operations; or

(3) Use of visual inspection to conduct a 100-percent examination for correct labeling during or after completion of finishing operations for hand-applied labeling. Such examination shall be performed by one person and independently verified by a second person.

(4) Use of any automated technique, including differentiation by labeling size and shape, that physically prevents incorrect labeling from being processed by labeling and packaging equipment.

(h) Printing devices on, or associated with, manufacturing lines used to imprint labeling upon the drug product unit label or case shall be monitored to assure that all imprinting conforms to the print specified in the batch production record.

Sec. 211.125 Labeling issuance.

(a) Strict control shall be exercised over labeling issued for use in drug product labeling operations.

(b) Labeling materials issued for a batch shall be carefully examined for identity and conformity to the labeling specified in the master or batch production records.

(c) Procedures shall be used to reconcile the quantities of labeling issued, used, and returned, and shall require evaluation of discrepancies found between the quantity of drug product finished and the quantity of labeling issued when such discrepancies are outside narrow preset limits based on historical operating data. Such discrepancies shall be investigated in accordance with 211.192. Labeling reconciliation is waived for cut or roll labeling if a 100-percent examination for correct labeling is performed in accordance with 211.122(g)(2).

(d) All excess labeling bearing lot or control numbers shall be destroyed.

(e) Returned labeling shall be maintained and stored in a manner to prevent mixups and provide proper identification.

(f) Procedures shall be written describing in sufficient detail the control procedures employed for the issuance of labeling; such written procedures shall be followed.

Sec. 211.130 Packaging and labeling operations.

There shall be written procedures designed to assure that correct labels, labeling, and packaging materials are used for drug products; such written procedures shall be followed. These procedures shall incorporate the following features:

(a) Prevention of mixups and cross-contamination by physical or spatial separation from operations on other drug products.

(b) Identification and handling of filled drug product containers that are set aside and held in unlabeled condition for future labeling operations to preclude mislabeling of individual containers, lots, or portions of lots. Identification need not be applied to each individual container but shall be sufficient to determine name, strength, quantity of contents, and lot or control number of each container.

(c) Identification of the drug product with a lot or control number that permits determination of the history of the manufacture and control of the batch.

(d) Examination of packaging and labeling materials for suitability and correctness before packaging operations, and documentation of such examination in the batch production record.

(e) Inspection of the packaging and labeling facilities immediately before use to assure that all drug products have been removed from previous operations. Inspection shall also be made to assure that packaging and labeling materials not suitable for subsequent operations have been removed. Results of inspection shall be documented in the batch production records.

Sec. 211.132 Tamper-evident packaging requirements for over-the-counter (OTC) human drug products.

(a) General. The Food and Drug Administration has the authority under the Federal Food, Drug, and Cosmetic Act (the act) to establish a uniform national requirement for tamper-evident packaging of OTC drug products that will improve the security of OTC drug packaging and help assure the safety and effectiveness of OTC drug products. An OTC drug product (except a dermatological, dentifrice, insulin, or lozenge product) for retail sale that is not packaged in a tam*per-resistant package or that is not pro*perly labeled under this section is adulterated under section 501 of the act or misbranded under section 502 of the act, or both.

(b) Requirements for tamper-evident package. (1) Each manufacturer and packer who packages an OTC drug product (except a dermatological, dentifrice, insulin, or lozenge product) for retail sale shall package the product in a tamper-evident package, if this product is accessible to the public while held for sale. A tamper-evident package is one having one or more indicators or barriers to entry which, if breached or missing, can reasonably be expected to provide visible evidence to consumers that tampering has occurred. To reduce the likelihood of successful tampering and to increase the likelihood that consumers will discover if a product has been tampered with, the package is required to be distinctive by design or by the use of one or more indicators or barriers to entry that employ an identifying characteristic (e.g., a pattern, name, registered trademark, logo, or picture). For purposes of this section, the term "distinctive by design" means the packaging cannot be duplicated with commonly available materials or through commonly available processes. A tamper-evident package may involve an immediate-container and closure system or secondary-container or carton system or any combination of systems intended to provide a visual indication of package integrity. The tamper-evident feature shall be designed to and shall remain intact when handled in a reasonable manner during manufacture, distribution, and retail display.

(2) In addition to the tamper-evident packaging feature *described* in paragraph (b)(1) of this section, any two-piece, hard gelatin capsule covered by this section must be sealed using an acceptable tamper-evident technology.

(c) Labeling. (1) In order to alert consumers to the specific tamper-evident feature(s) used, each retail package of an OTC drug product covered by this section (except ammonia inhalant in crushable glass ampules, containers of compressed medical oxygen, or aerosol products that depend upon the power of a liquefied or compressed gas to expel the contents from the container) is required to bear a statement that:

(i) Identifies all tamper-evident feature(s) and any capsule sealing technologies used to comply with paragraph (b) of this section;

(ii) Is prominently placed on the package; and

(iii) Is so placed that it will be unaffected if the tamper-evident feature of the package is breached or missing.

(2) If the tamper-evident feature chosen to meet the requirements in paragraph (b) of this section uses an identifying characteristic, that characteristic is required to be referred to in *the labeling statement. For example, the labeling statement on* a bottle with a shrink band could say "For your protection, this bottle has an imprinted seal around the neck."

(d) Request for exemptions from packaging and labeling requirements. A manufacturer or packer may request an exemption from the packaging and labeling requirements of this section. A request for an exemption is required to be submitted in the form of a citizen petition under 10.30 of this chapter and should be clearly identified on the envelope as a "Request for Exemption from the Tamper-Evident Packaging Rule." The petition is required to contain the following:

(1) The name of the drug product or, if the petition seeks an exemption for a drug class, the name of the drug class, and a list of products within that class.

(2) The reasons that the drug product's compliance with the tamper-evident packaging or labeling requirements of this section is unnecessary or cannot be achieved.

(3) A description of alternative steps that are available, or that the *petitioner has already taken, to reduce the likelihood that* the product or drug class will be the subject of malicious adulteration.

(4) Other information justifying an exemption.

(e) OTC drug products subject to approved new drug applications. Holders of approved new drug applications for OTC drug products are required under 314.70 of this chapter to provide the agency with notification of changes in packaging and labeling to comply with the requirements of this section. Changes in packaging and labeling required by this regulation may be made *before FDA approval, as provided under* 314.70(c) of this chapter. Manufacturing changes by which capsules are to be sealed require prior FDA approval under 314.70(b) of this chapter.

(f) Poison Prevention Packaging Act of 1970. This section does not affect any requirements for "special packaging" as defined under 310.3 (l) of this chapter and required under the Poison Prevention Packaging Act of 1970.

Sec. 211.134 Drug product inspection.

(a) Packaged and labeled products shall be examined during finishing operations to provide assurance that containers and packages in the lot have the correct label.

(b) A representative sample of units shall be collected at the completion of finishing operations and shall be visually examined for correct labeling.

(c) Results of these examinations shall be recorded in the batch production or control records.

Sec. 211.137 Expiration dating.

(a) To assure that a drug product meets applicable standards of identity, strength, quality, and purity at the time of use, it shall bear an expiration date determined by appropriate stability testing described in 211.166.

(b) Expiration dates shall be related to any storage conditions stated on the labeling, as determined by stability studies described in 211.166.

(c) If the drug product is to be reconstituted at the time of dispensing, its labeling shall bear expiration information for both the reconstituted and unreconstituted drug products.

(d) Expiration dates shall appear on labeling in accordance with the requirements of 201.17 of this chapter.

(e) Homeopathic drug products shall be exempt from the requirements of this section.

(f) Allergenic extracts that are labeled "No U.S. Standard of Potency" are exempt from the requirements of this section.

(g) New drug products for investigational use are exempt from the requirements of this section, provided that they meet appropriate standards or specifications as demonstrated by stability studies during their use in clinical investigations. Where new drug products for investigational use are to be reconstituted at the time of dispensing, their labeling shall bear expiration information for the reconstituted drug product.

(h) Pending consideration of a proposed exemption, published in the Federal Register of September 29, 1978, the requirements in this section shall not be enforced for human OTC drug products if their labeling does not bear dosage limitations and they are stable for at least 3 years as supported by appropriate stability data.

Subpart H--Holding and Distribution

Sec. 211.142 Warehousing procedures.

Written procedures describing the warehousing of drug products shall be established and followed. They shall include:

(a) Quarantine of drug products before release by the quality control unit.

(b) Storage of drug products under appropriate conditions of temperature, humidity, and light so that the identity, strength, quality, and purity of the drug products are not affected.

Sec. 211.150 Distribution procedures.

Written procedures shall be established, and followed, describing the distribution of drug products. They shall include:

(a) A procedure whereby the oldest approved stock of a drug product is distributed first. Deviation from this requirement is permitted if such deviation is temporary and appropriate.

(b) A system by which the distribution of each lot of drug product can be readily determined to facilitate its recall if necessary.

Subpart I--Laboratory Controls

Sec. 211.160 General requirements.

(a) The establishment of any specifications, standards, sampling plans, test procedures, or other laboratory control mechanisms required by this subpart, including any change in such specifications, standards, sampling plans, test procedures, or other laboratory control mechanisms, shall be drafted by the appropriate organizational unit and reviewed and approved by the quality control unit. The requirements in this subpart shall be followed and shall be documented at the time of performance. Any deviation from the written specifications, standards, sampling plans, test procedures, or other laboratory control mechanisms shall be recorded and justified.

(b) Laboratory controls shall include the establishment of scientifically sound and appropriate specifications, standards, sampling plans, and test procedures designed to assure that components, drug product containers, closures, in-process materials, labeling, and drug products conform to appropriate standards of identity, strength, quality, and purity. Laboratory controls shall include:

(1) Determination of conformity to applicable written specifications for the acceptance of each lot within each shipment of components, drug product containers, closures, and labeling used in the manufacture, processing, packing, or holding of drug products. The specifications shall include a description of the sampling and testing procedures used. Samples shall be representative and adequately identified. Such procedures shall also require appropriate retesting of any component, drug product container, or closure that is subject to deterioration.

(2) Determination of conformance to written specifications and a description of sampling and testing procedures for in-process materials. Such samples shall be representative and properly identified.

(3) Determination of conformance to written descriptions of sampling procedures and appropriate specifications for drug products. Such samples shall be representative and properly identified.

(4) The calibration of instruments, apparatus, gauges, and recording devices at suitable intervals in accordance with an established written program containing specific directions, schedules, limits for accuracy and precision, and provisions for remedial action in the event accuracy and/or precision limits are not met. Instruments, apparatus, gauges, and recording devices not meeting established specifications shall not be used.

Sec. 211.165 Testing and release for distribution.

(a) For each batch of drug product, there shall be appropriate laboratory determination of satisfactory conformance to final specifications for the drug product, including the identity and strength of each active ingredient, prior to release. Where sterility and/or pyrogen testing are conducted on specific batches of shortlived radiopharmaceuticals, such batches may be released prior to completion of sterility and/or pyrogen testing, provided such testing is completed as soon as possible.

(b) There shall be appropriate laboratory testing, as necessary, of each batch of drug product required to be free of objectionable microorganisms.

(c) Any sampling and testing plans shall be described in written procedures that shall include the method of sampling and the number of units per batch to be tested; such written procedure shall be followed.

(d) Acceptance criteria for the sampling and testing conducted by the quality control unit shall be adequate to assure that batches of drug products meet each appropriate specification and appropriate statistical quality control criteria as a condition for their approval and release. The statistical quality control criteria shall include appropriate acceptance levels and/or appropriate rejection levels.

(e) The accuracy, sensitivity, specificity, and reproducibility of test methods employed by the firm shall be established and documented.

Such validation and documentation may be accomplished in accordance with 211.194(a)(2).

(f) Drug products failing to meet established standards or specifications and any other relevant quality control criteria shall be rejected. Reprocessing may be performed. Prior to acceptance and use, reprocessed material must meet appropriate standards, specifications, and any other relevant critieria.

Sec. 211.166 Stability testing.

(a) There shall be a written testing program designed to assess the stability characteristics of drug products. The results of such stability testing shall be used in determining appropriate storage conditions and expiration dates. The written program shall be followed and shall include:

(1) Sample size and test intervals based on statistical criteria for each attribute examined to assure valid estimates of stability;

(2) Storage conditions for samples retained for testing;

(3) Reliable, meaningful, and specific test methods;

(4) Testing of the drug product in the same container-closure system as that in which the drug product is marketed;

(5) Testing of drug products for reconstitution at the time of dispensing (as directed in the labeling) as well as after they are reconstituted.

(b) An adequate number of batches of each drug product shall be tested to determine an appropriate expiration date and a record of such data shall be maintained. Accelerated studies, combined with basic stability information on the components, drug products, and container-closure system, may be used to support tentative expiration dates provided full shelf life studies are not available and are being conducted. Where data from accelerated studies are used to project a tentative expiration date that is beyond a date supported by actual shelf life studies, there must be stability studies conducted, including drug product testing at appropriate intervals, until the tentative expiration date is verified or the appropriate expiration date determined.

(c) For homeopathic drug products, the requirements of this section are as follows:

(1) There shall be a written assessment of stability based at least on testing or examination of the drug product for compatibility of the ingredients, and based on marketing experience with the drug product to indicate that there is no degradation of the product for the normal or expected period of use.

(2) Evaluation of stability shall be based on the same container-closure system in which the drug product is being marketed.

(d) Allergenic extracts that are labeled "No U.S. Standard of Potency" are exempt from the requirements of this section.

Sec. 211.167 Special testing requirements.

(a) For each batch of drug product purporting to be sterile and/or pyrogen-free, there shall be appropriate laboratory testing to determine conformance to such requirements. The test procedures shall be in writing and shall be followed.

(b) For each batch of ophthalmic ointment, there shall be appropriate testing to determine conformance to specifications regarding the presence of foreign particles and harsh or abrasive substances. The test procedures shall be in writing and shall be followed.

(c) For each batch of controlled-release dosage form, there shall be appropriate laboratory testing to determine conformance to the specifications for the rate of release of each active ingredient. The test procedures shall be in writing and shall be followed.

Sec. 211.170 Reserve samples.

(a) An appropriately identified reserve sample that is representative of each lot in each shipment of each active ingredient shall be retained. The reserve sample consists of at least twice the quantity necessary for all tests required to determine whether the active ingredient meets its established specifications, except for sterility and pyrogen testing. The retention time is as follows:

(1) For an active ingredient in a drug product other than those described in paragraphs (a) (2) and (3) of this section, the reserve

sample shall be retained for 1 year after the expiration date of the last lot of the drug product containing the active ingredient.

(2) For an active ingredient in a radioactive drug product, except for nonradioactive reagent kits, the reserve sample shall be retained for:

(i) Three months after the expiration date of the last lot of the drug product containing the active ingredient if the expiration dating period of the drug product is 30 days or less; or

(ii) Six months after the expiration date of the last lot of the drug product containing the active ingredient if the expiration dating period of the drug product is more than 30 days.

(3) For an active ingredient in an OTC drug product that is exempt from bearing an expiration date under 211.137, the reserve sample shall be retained for 3 years after distribution of the last lot of the drug product containing the active ingredient.

(b) An appropriately identified reserve sample that is representative of each lot or batch of drug product shall be retained and stored under conditions consistent with product labeling. The reserve sample shall be stored in the same immediate container-closure system in which the drug product is marketed or in one that has essentially the same characteristics. The reserve sample consists of at least twice the quantity necessary to perform all the required tests, except those for sterility and pyrogens. Except for those for drug products described in paragraph (b)(2) of this section, reserve samples from representative sample lots or batches selected by acceptable statistical procedures shall be examined visually at least once a year for evidence of deterioration unless visual examination would affect the integrity of the reserve sample. Any evidence of reserve sample deterioration shall be investigated in accordance with 211.192. The results of the examination shall be recorded and maintained with other stability data on the drug product. Reserve samples of compressed medical gases need not be retained. The retention time is as follows:

(1) For a drug product other than those described in paragraphs (b) (2) and (3) of this section, the reserve sample shall be retained for 1 year after the expiration date of the drug product.

(2) For a radioactive drug product, except for nonradioactive reagent kits, the reserve sample shall be retained for:

(i) Three months after the expiration date of the drug product if the expiration dating period of the drug product is 30 days or less; or

(ii) Six months after the expiration date of the drug product if the expiration dating period of the drug product is more than 30 days.

(3) For an OTC drug product that is exempt for bearing an expiration date under 211.137, the reserve sample must be retained for 3 years after the lot or batch of drug product is distributed.

Sec. 211.173 Laboratory animals.

Animals used in testing components, in-process materials, or drug products for compliance with established specifications shall be maintained and controlled in a manner that assures their suitability for their intended use. They shall be identified, and adequate records shall be maintained showing the history of their use.

Sec. 211.176 Penicillin contamination.

If a reasonable possibility exists that a non-penicillin drug product has been exposed to cross-contamination with penicillin, the non-penicillin drug product shall be tested for the presence of penicillin. Such drug product shall not be marketed if detectable levels are found when tested according to procedures specified in 'Procedures for Detecting and Measuring Penicillin Contamination in Drugs,' which is incorporated by reference. Copies are available from the Division of Research and Testing (HFD-470), Center for Drug Evaluation and Research, Food and *Drug Administration, 5100 Paint Branch Pkwy., College Park, MD 20740, or available fo*r inspection at the National Archives and Records Administration (NARA). For information on the availability of this material at NARA, call 202-741-6030, or go to: http://www.archives.gov/federal_register/code_of_federal_regulations/ibr_locations.html.

Subpart J--Records and Reports

Sec. 211.180 General requirements.

(a) Any production, control, or distribution record that is required to be maintained in compliance with this part and is specifically associated with a batch of a drug product shall be retained for at least 1 year after the expiration date of the batch or, in the case of certain OTC drug products lacking expiration dating because they meet the criteria for exemption under 211.137, 3 years after distribution of the batch.

(b) Records shall be maintained for all components, drug product containers, closures, and labeling for at least 1 year after the expiration date or, in the case of certain OTC drug products lacking expiration dating because they meet the criteria for exemption under 211.137, 3 years after distribution of the last lot of drug product incorporating the component or using the container, closure, or labeling.

(c) All records required under this part, or copies of such records, shall be readily available for authorized inspection during the retention period at the establishment where the activities described in such records occurred. These records or copies thereof shall be subject to photocopying or other means of reproduction as part of such inspection. Records that can be immediately retrieved from another location by computer or other electronic means shall be considered as meeting the requirements of this paragraph.

(d) Records required under this part may be retained either as original records or as true copies such as photocopies, microfilm, microfiche, or other accurate reproductions of the original records. Where reduction techniques, such as microfilming, are used, suitable reader and photocopying equipment shall be readily available.

(e) Written records required by this part shall be maintained so that data therein can be used for evaluating, at least annually, the quality standards of each drug product to determine the need for changes in drug product specifications or manufacturing or control procedures. Written procedures shall be established and followed for such evaluations and shall include provisions for:

(1) A review of a representative number of batches, whether approved or rejected, and, where applicable, records associated with the batch.

(2) A review of complaints, recalls, returned or salvaged drug products, and investigations conducted under 211.192 for each drug product.

(f) Procedures shall be established to assure that the responsible officials of the firm, if they are not personally involved in or immediately aware of such actions, are notified in writing of any investigations conducted under 211.198, 211.204, or 211.208 of these regulations, any recalls, reports of inspectional observations issued by the Food and Drug Administration, or any regulatory actions relating to good manufacturing practices brought by the Food and Drug Administration.

Sec. 211.182 Equipment cleaning and use log.

A written record of major equipment cleaning, maintenance (except routine maintenance such as lubrication and adjustments), and use shall be included in individual equipment logs that show the date, time, product, and lot number of each batch processed. If equipment is dedicated to manufacture of one product, then individual equipment logs are not required, provided that lots or batches of such product follow in numerical order and are manufactured in numerical sequence. In cases where dedicated equipment is employed, the records of cleaning, maintenance, and use shall be part of the batch record. The persons performing and double-checking the cleaning and maintenance (or, if the cleaning and maintenance is performed using automated equipment under 211.68, just the person verifying the cleaning and maintenance done by the automated equipment) shall date and sign or initial the log indicating that the work was performed. Entries in the log shall be in chronological order.

Sec. 211.184 Component, drug product container, closure, and labeling records.

These records shall include the following:

(a) The identity and quantity of each shipment of each lot of components, drug product containers, closures, and labeling; the name of the supplier; the supplier's lot number(s) if known; the receiving code as specified in 211.80; and the date of receipt. The name and location of the prime manufacturer, if different from the supplier, shall be listed if known.

(b) The results of any test or examination performed (including those performed as required by 211.82(a), 211.84(d), or 211.122(a)) and the conclusions derived therefrom.

(c) An individual inventory record of each component, drug product container, and closure and, for each component, a reconciliation of the use of each lot of such component. The inventory record shall contain sufficient information to allow determination of any batch or lot of drug product associated with the use of each component, drug product container, and closure.

(d) Documentation of the examination and review of labels and labeling for conformity with established specifications in accord with 211.122(c) and 211.130(c).

(e) The disposition of rejected components, drug product containers, closure, and labeling.

Sec. 211.186 Master production and control records.

(a) To assure uniformity from batch to batch, master production and control records for each drug product, including each batch size thereof, shall be prepared, dated, and signed (full signature, handwritten) by one person and independently checked, dated, and signed by a second person. The preparation of master production and control records shall be described in a written procedure and such written procedure shall be followed.

(b) Master production and control records shall include:

(1) The name and strength of the product and a description of the dosage form;

(2) The name and weight or measure of each active ingredient per dosage unit or per unit of weight or measure of the drug product, and a statement of the total weight or measure of any dosage unit;

(3) A complete list of components designated by names or codes sufficiently specific to indicate any special quality characteristic;

(4) An accurate statement of the weight or measure of each component, using the same weight system (metric, avoirdupois, or apothecary) for each component. Reasonable variations may be permitted, however, in the amount of components necessary for the preparation in the dosage form, provided they are justified in the master production and control records;

(5) A statement concerning any calculated excess of component;

(6) A statement of theoretical weight or measure at appropriate phases of processing;

(7) A statement of theoretical yield, including the maximum and minimum percentages of theoretical yield beyond which investigation according to 211.192 is required;

(8) A description of the drug product containers, closures, and packaging materials, including a specimen or copy of each label and all other labeling signed and dated by the person or persons responsible for approval of such labeling;

(9) Complete manufacturing and control instructions, sampling and testing procedures, specifications, special notations, and precautions to be followed.

Sec. 211.188 Batch production and control records.

Batch production and control records shall be prepared for each batch of drug product produced and shall include complete information relating to the production and control of each batch. These records shall include:

(a) An accurate reproduction of the appropriate master production or control record, checked for accuracy, dated, and signed;

(b) Documentation that each significant step in the manufacture, processing, packing, or holding of the batch was accomplished, including:

(1) Dates;

(2) Identity of individual major equipment and lines used;

(3) Specific identification of each batch of component or in-process material used;

(4) Weights and measures of components used in the course of processing;

(5) In-process and laboratory control results;

(6) Inspection of the packaging and labeling area before and after use;

(7) A statement of the actual yield and a statement of the percentage of theoretical yield at appropriate phases of processing;

(8) Complete labeling control records, including specimens or copies of all labeling used;

(9) Description of drug product containers and closures;

(10) Any sampling performed;

(11) Identification of the persons performing and directly supervising or checking each significant step in the operation, or if a significant step in the operation is performed by automated equipment under 211.68, the identification of the person checking the significant step performed by the automated equipment.

(12) Any investigation made according to 211.192.

(13) Results of examinations made in accordance with 211.134.

Sec. 211.192 Production record review.

All drug product production and control records, including those for packaging and labeling, shall be reviewed and approved by the quality control unit to determine compliance with all established, approved written procedures before a batch is released or distributed. Any unexplained discrepancy (including a percentage of theoretical yield exceeding the maximum or minimum percentages established in master production and control records) or the failure of a batch or any of its components to meet any of its specifications shall be thoroughly investigated, whether or not the batch has already been distributed. The investigation shall extend to other batches of the same drug product and other drug products that may have been associated with the specific failure or discrepancy. A written record of the investigation shall be made and shall include the conclusions and followup.

Sec. 211.194 Laboratory records.

(a) Laboratory records shall include complete data derived from all tests necessary to assure compliance with established specifications and standards, including examinations and assays, as follows:

(1) A description of the sample received for testing with identification of source (that is, location from where sample was obtained),

quantity, lot number or other distinctive code, date sample was taken, and date sample was received for testing.

(2) A statement of each method used in the testing of the sample. The statement shall indicate the location of data that establish that the methods used in the testing of the sample meet proper standards of accuracy and reliability as applied to the product tested. (If the method employed is in the current revision of the United States Pharmacopeia, National Formulary, AOAC INTERNATIONAL, Book of Methods, 1 or in other recognized standard references, or is detailed in an approved new drug application and the referenced method is not modified, a statement indicating the method and reference will suffice). The suitability of all testing methods used shall be verified under actual conditions of use.

(3) A statement of the weight or measure of sample used for each test, where appropriate.

(4) A complete record of all data secured in the course of each test, including all graphs, charts, and spectra from laboratory instrumentation, properly identified to show the specific component, drug product container, closure, in-process material, or drug product, and lot tested.

(5) A record of all calculations performed in connection with the test, including units of measure, conversion factors, and equivalency factors.

(6) A statement of the results of tests and how the results compare with established standards of identity, strength, quality, and purity for the component, drug product container, closure, in-process material, or drug product tested.

(7) The initials or signature of the person who performs each test and the date(s) the tests were performed.

(8) The initials or signature of a second person showing that the original records have been reviewed for accuracy, completeness, and compliance with established standards.

(b) Complete records shall be maintained of any modification of an established method employed in testing. Such records shall include the reason for the modification and data to verify that the modification produced results that are at least as accurate and reliable for the material being tested as the established method.

(c) Complete records shall be maintained of any testing and standardization of laboratory reference standards, reagents, and standard solutions.

(d) Complete records shall be maintained of the periodic calibration of laboratory instruments, apparatus, gauges, and recording devices required by 211.160(b)(4).

(e) Complete records shall be maintained of all stability testing performed in accordance with 211.166.

1 Copies may be obtained from: AOAC INTERNATIONAL, 481 North Frederick Ave., suite 500, Gaithersburg, MD 20877.

Sec. 211.196 Distribution records.

Distribution records shall contain the name and strength of the product and description of the dosage form, name and address of the consignee, date and quantity shipped, and lot or control number of the drug product. For compressed medical gas products, distribution records are not required to contain lot or control numbers.

Sec. 211.198 Complaint files.

(a) Written procedures describing the handling of all written and oral complaints regarding a drug product shall be established and followed. Such procedures shall include provisions for review by the quality control unit, of any complaint involving the possible failure of a drug product to meet any of its specifications and, for such drug products, a determination as to the need for an investigation in accordance with 211.192. Such procedures shall include provisions for review to determine whether the complaint represents a serious and unexpected adverse drug experience which is required to be reported to the Food and Drug Administration in accordance with 310.305 and 514.80 of this chapter.

(b) A written record of each complaint shall be maintained in a file designated for drug product complaints. The file regarding such drug product complaints shall be maintained at the establishment where the drug product involved was manufactured, processed, or packed, or such file may be maintained at another facility if the written records in such files are readily available for inspection at that other facility. Written records involving a drug product shall be maintained until at least 1 year after the expiration date of the drug product, or 1 year after the date that the complaint was received, whichever is longer. In the case of certain OTC drug products lacking expiration dating because they meet the criteria for exemption under 211.137, such written records shall be maintained for 3 years after distribution of the drug product.

(1) The written record shall include the following information, where known: the name and strength of the drug product, lot number, name of complainant, nature of complaint, and reply to complainant.

(2) Where an investigation under 211.192 is conducted, the written record shall include the findings of the investigation and followup. The record or copy of the record of the investigation shall be maintained at the establishment where the investigation occurred in accordance with 211.180(c).

(3) Where an investigation under 211.192 is not conducted, the written record shall include the reason that an investigation was found not to be necessary and the name of the responsible person making such a determination.

Subpart K--Returned and Salvaged Drug Products

Sec. 211.204 Returned drug products.

Returned drug products shall be identified as such and held. If the conditions under which returned drug products have been held, stored, or shipped before or during their return, or if the condition of the drug product, its container, carton, or labeling, as a result of storage or shipping, casts doubt on the safety, identity, strength, quality or purity of the drug product, the returned drug product shall be destroyed unless examination, testing, or other investigations prove the drug product meets appropriate standards of safety, identity, strength, quality, or purity. A drug product may be reprocessed provided the subsequent drug product meets appropriate standards, specifications, and characteristics. Records of returned drug products shall be maintained and shall include the name and label potency of the drug product dosage form, lot number (or control number or batch number), reason for the return, quantity returned, date of disposition, and ultimate disposition of the returned drug product. If the reason for a drug product being returned implicates associated batches, an appropriate investigation shall be conducted in accordance with the requirements of 211.192. Procedures for the holding, testing, and reprocessing of returned drug products shall be in writing and shall be followed.

Sec. 211.208 Drug product salvaging.

Drug products that have been subjected to improper storage conditions including extremes in temperature, humidity, smoke, fumes, pressure, age, or radiation due to natural disasters, fires, accidents, or equipment failures shall not be salvaged and returned to the marketplace. Whenever there is a question whether drug products have been subjected to such conditions, salvaging operations may be conducted only if there is (a) evidence from laboratory tests and assays (including animal feeding studies where applicable) that the drug products meet all applicable standards of identity, strength, quality, and purity and (b) evidence from inspection of the premises that the drug products and their associated packaging were not subjected to improper storage conditions as a result of the disaster or accident. Organoleptic examinations shall be acceptable only as supplemental evidence that the drug products meet appropriate standards of identity, strength, quality, and purity. Records including name, lot number, and disposition shall be maintained for drug products subject to this section.

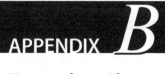

Example—Short Change Control Form

SHORT CHANGE CONTROL FORM

DATE:

Section A

Project #:		Change Number
Controlled Item		Item Version
Identification of Aspect to be Change	For Document give section number / page number For Software give Module, Screen or Report name	

Change Details

Include indication of
importance and urgency

Tick if Continued Overleaf ☐ ✎

Change Requested by:		Date:
Print Name		

Section B

Primary Investigator	
Impact, give details of other items affected	

Investigation Outcome Reject / Action at No Cost / Action at Cost	Suggested Priority High / Medium / Low	Date

Section C

Validation Review:		Date
Disposition:		
Engineering Review:		
Disposition		
Other Review (Dept.):		
Disposition		
QA Review:		
Disposition		

SHORT CHANGE CONTROL FORM

DOCUMENT CONTROL

Title:
Issue:
Date:
Author:
Distribution:

Reference:
Filename:
Control: Reissue as complete document only

Change :

APPROVED   ☐

REJECTED   ☐

DOCUMENT SIGNOFF

Nature of Signoff	Person	Signature	Date	Role
Author				Senior Consultant
Reviewer				Project Controller

DOCUMENT CHANGE RECORD

Date	Version	Author	Change Details
	Issue 1 Draft 1		Initial Draft
	Issue 1 Draft 2		Update following XX review comments
	Issue 1 Draft 3		Re-formatting
	Issue 1		Add Introduction and issue

Additional ICH and FDA Guidelines

IMPORTANT ICH AND FDA GUIDELINES

ICH (NOTE: Some of the categories have additional documents. These can be found on ICH.org)

Q1—Stability Testing
  Q1A—Stability Testing of New Drug Substances and Products
  Q1C—Stability Testing New Dosage Forms
  Q1E—Evaluation of Stability Data
Q2—Validation of Analytical Procedures: Text and Methodology
Q3—Impurities
  Q3A—Impurities in New Drug Substances
  Q3B—Impurities in New Drug Products
  Q3C—Impurities: Guideline for Residual Solvents
Q4—Pharmacopoeias
  Q4B Annex 5—Disintegration Test General Chapter
  Q4B Annex 7—Dissolution Test General Chapter
  Q4B Annex 8—Sterility Test General Chapter
  Q4B Annex 9—Tablet Friability General Chapter
Q5—Quality of Biological Products
  Q5A—Viral Safety of Biotechnology Products Derived from Cell Lines of Human or Animal Origin
  Q5C—Stability Testing of Biotechnology/Biological Products
Q6—Specifications
  Q6A—Test Procedures and Acceptance Criteria for New Drug Substances and New Drug Products
  Q6B—Test Procedures and Acceptance Criteria for Biotechnology/Biological Products
Q7—Good Manufacturing Guideline for Active Pharmaceutical Ingredients
Q8—Pharmaceutical Development
Q9—Quality Risk Management

Q10—Pharmaceutical Quality Systems
Q11—Development of Manufacture of Drug Substances
Q12—Technical and Regulatory Considerations for Pharmaceutical Product Lifecycle Management

FDA Guidelines (NOTE: Several ICH guidelines are also FDA guidelines, additional FDA guidelines can be found on fda.gov)

Current good Manufacturing Practice for Phase 1 Investigational New Drugs

Investigating Out-of-Specification Test Results for Pharmaceutical Production

PAT—A Framework for Innovative Pharmaceutical Development, Manufacturing, and Quality Assurance

Preparation of Investigational New Drug Products (Human and Animal)

Process Validation: General Principles and Practices

Quality System Approach to Pharmaceutical Current Good Manufacturing Practice Regulations

Sterile Drug Products Produced by Aseptic Processing—Current Good Manufacturing Practice

Current Good Manufacturing Practice—Interim Guidance for Human Drug Compounding Outsourcing Facilities Under Section 503B of the FD & C Act

Current Good Manufacturing Practice Requirements for Combination Products

Note: Page numbers followed by "f" and "t" refer to figures and tables, respectively.

A

Active pharmaceutical ingredient (API), 37, 59, 91–93
  pre-market approval, 29
  process installation, 28–29
Air filtration, 25–26, 157–158
Air heating, 25–26, 157–158
American Society for Testing and Materials (ASTM), 30
Annual Product Reports (APRs), 10, 37, 39–41
Annual product review, 121–123, 126
Automatic equipment, 22–24, 160–161

B

Basic equipment and utility qualification, 59, 64f
  commissioning, 60–62
  Installation Qualification, 64–67, 65t
  laboratory Equipment Qualification, 67–68
  level of qualification, determining, 60
  Operational Qualification, 64–67, 66t
  Performance Qualification, 67, 67t
  qualification protocol execution, 68–70, 68t
    calibration, 69–70
    preventive maintenance programs, 69–70
    reports, 69
Batch production and control records, 27–28
  general requirements, 28
  person identification on, 29
Batch production and control records, 185–186
Black box testing, 74
Building Management Systems (BMS), 83–84
Buildings and facilities, for CGMPs, 156
  air filtration, 157–158
  air heating, 157–158
  cooling, 157–158
  design and construction features, 156–157
  lighting, 157
  maintenance, 159
  plumbing, 158
  sanitation, 158–159
  sewage and refuse, 158
  ventilation, 157–158
  washing and toilet facilities, 158

C

Calibration, 69–70
Certified quality audit (CQA), 37
Change control, 125
  process, 40–41
  role in process validation, 35–37
Charge-in of components, 166–167
Clean in Place (CIP), 138–139
Cleaning, 136
  equipment, 138–139
  facility design and, 137–138
  general considerations for, 136–137
  sampling method and, 139–140
  validation, 5–6
Closures, 162, 165
  approval or rejection of, 24–25, 162–164
  general requirements, 162
  records and reports, 183–184
  rejected, 165
  retesting of approved, 165
  testing of, 24–25, 162–164
  untested, receipt and storage of, 162
  use of approved, 164
Code of Federal Regulations (CFR), 6–7, 33, 59, 62–63, 153
  Title 21, 15, 17
Commissioning, 60–62
Complaint files, 188–189
Compliance Program Guidance (CPG), 28
  API process installation, 28–29
  APIs subject to pre-market approval, 29
  computerized drug processing.
    See Computerized drug processing
  input/output checking, 29
  process validation requirements, for drug products, 29
Components
  approval or rejection of, 24–25
  control, 162

Components (*Continued*)
  approval or rejection of, 162–164
  approved components, retesting of, 165
  approved components, use of, 164
  general requirements, 162
  records and reports, 183–184
  rejected components, 165
  testing of components, 162–164
  untested components, receipt and storage
      of, 162
  testing of, 24–25
Computer systems validation (CSV), 71–74
  black box testing, 74
  grey box testing, 74
  white box testing, 74
Computerized drug processing, 29
  CGMP applicability to hardware and
      software, 29
  person identification on batch production
      and control records, 29
  source code for process control application
      programs, 29
Computers and automated systems, 71
  distributed control system, 83–84, 84*t*
  general documentation, 73–78, 73*t*
  general testing, 73–78
  Installation Qualification, 75–77, 77*t*
  microprocessors, 79
  networks, 82, 82*t*
  Operational Qualification, 75–76, 78*t*
  Performance Qualification, 78, 78*t*
  personal computers, 81, 82*t*
  programmed logic controllers, 80–81, 81*t*
  qualification testing program, 74–78
  Supervisory Control and Data Acquisition,
      83, 83*t*
Concurrent validation, 7
Construction features, 25
Consultants, 156
Continued process verification (CPV), 10, 104,
      121–123, 125–126, 136
  annual product reviews, 126
  change control, 125
  process metrics, 125
  trend analysis, 125
Control charts, 126–129, 127*f*, 127*t*, 128*f*
Control limits (CL), 99
Cooling, 25–26, 157–158
Corrective action and/or a preventative action
      (CAPA), 116
Critical Process Parameters (CPPs), 8, 92–93,
      97–98, 99*t*, 104, 106, 111, 121–122,
      125

Critical Quality Attributes (CQAs), 8, 12, 92,
      97–98, 99*t*, 104, 111, 121–122, 125–126
Current Good Manufacturing Practices
      (CGMPs), 4–7, 12, 33–35, 51–53,
      62–63, 133. *See also* Good
      Manufacturing Practices (GMPs)
  applicability to hardware and software, 29
  for finished pharmaceuticals
    buildings and facilities, 156
    closures, 162
    components control, 162
    drug product containers, 162
    equipment, 159
    general provisions, 153
    holding and distribution, 175
    laboratory controls, 176
    organization and personnel, 154
    packaging and labeling control, 169
    productions and process control, 165
    records and reports, 181
    returned and salvaged drug products, 189

D

Deficiencies, 113
Design features, 25
Design Specifications (DS), 35
Deviations, 113, 165–166
  classification, decision tree for, 116*f*
  critical, 115
  investigation, 117
  level of, 115
  root cause of, 117
Distributed control system (DCS), 83–84, 84*t*
Distribution procedures, 175–176
Distribution records, 188
Drug product(s)
  containers, 162, 165
    approval or rejection of, 24–25, 162–164
    general requirements, 162
    records and reports, 183–184
    rejected, 165
    retesting of approved, 165
    testing of, 24–25, 162–164
    untested, receipt and storage of, 162
    use of approved, 164
  inspection, 174
  process validation requirements for, 29
  returned, 189–190
  salvaging, 190
  sampling and testing of, 167–168
  testing of, 18–21
    general requirements for, 20–21
    sampling of, 20–21

E

Edge of failure (EOF), 99
Electromagnetic Interference (EMI), 78*t*
Electronically Erasable Programmed Random Only Memory (EEPROM), 79
Electronically Programmed Random Only Memory (EPROM), 79
Electronic equipment, 22–24, 160–161
Enterprise Resource Planning (ERP), 83–84
Equipment, 159
  automatic, 22–24, 160–161
  cleaning, 138–139, 160, 183
  construction, 159–160
  design, 21–22, 159
  electronic, 22–24, 160–161
  filters, 161
  identification, 167
  location, 21–22, 159
  maintenance, 160
  mechanical, 22–24, 160–161
  size, 21–22, 159
Equipment Qualification (EQ), 65. *See also* Installation Qualification (IQ); Operational Qualification (OQ)
  laboratory, 67–68
Exceptions, 113
Expiration dating, 174–175

F

Facility design, and cleaning, 137–138
Facility qualification
  check list for, 135*t*
Factory Acceptance Test (FAT), 59–62
Failure Mode, Effect and Criticality Analysis (FMECA), 94
Failure Mode Effect Analysis (FMEA), 94, 95*f*, 96*f*, 97
Fault Tree Analysis (FTA), 94
FDA guidelines, 194
Filters, 161
Food, Drug, and Cosmetic Act (FD&C), 6–7, 15–17
Functional Requirements (FRS), 35

G

Gantt chart, 55–57, 56*f*
Good Automated Manufacturing Practice (GAMP), 71–72, 74–75, 80
Good Documentation Practices (GDPs), 111–112
Good Manufacturing Practices (GMPs), 3–4, 6, 15, 33–36, 39–41, 47–48, 51, 62, 64–65, 133. *See also* Current Good Manufacturing Practices (CGMPs)
Grey box testing, 74

H

Hardware
  CGMP applicability to, 29
  functional testing of, 78*t*
Hazard Analysis Critical Control Points (HACCP), 94
Hold times, 136–137
Human Machine Interface (HMI), 80

I

ICH Q9 approach, for risk assessment, 93, 93*f*
In-process materials, sampling and testing of, 21, 167–168
Input/output checking, 29
Installation Qualification (IQ), 36, 62, 64–67, 65*t*, 75–77
  computer physical components, 77*t*
  for process development, 101
  software structural testing, 77*t*
International Conference on Harmonization (ICH), 15–16
  guidelines, 193–194
  ICH Q9 approach, for risk assessment, 93, 93*f*
ISO room classifications, 135

L

Labeling
  control, 169
  issuance, 170–171
  operations, 171–172
Laboratory animals, 181
Laboratory controls, 176
  general requirements, 176–177
  laboratory animals, 181
  penicillin contamination, 181
  reserve samples, 179–181
  special testing requirements, 179
  stability testing, 178–179
  testing and release for distribution, 177–178
Laboratory records, 186–188
Ladder logic, 80
Legacy products, 7–9, 8*f*, 123–125
Level of qualification, determining, 60
Life cycle approach, 33–35, 34*f*
Lighting, 25, 157

M

Master production and control records, 26–27, 184–185
  general requirements, 28
Materials examination, 169–170
Materials Resource Planning Systems (MRP), 83–84

Mechanical equipment, 22–24, 160–161
Microbiological contamination, control of, 168–169
Microprocessors, 79
Mix-ups, prevention of, 25

N
Networks, 82
  qualification, 82*t*
Normal distribution, 127*f*
Normal operating range (NOR), 100, 104

O
Operational Qualification (OQ), 36, 62, 64–67, 66*t*, 75–76
  hardware and software, functional testing of, 78*t*
  for process development, 101
Out of Specification (OOS), 113
Over-the-counter (OTC) human drug products, tamper-evident packaging requirements for, 172–174

P
Packaging, 169
  drug product inspection, 174
  expiration dating, 174–175
  materials examination and usage criteria, 169–170
  operations, 171–172
  OTC human drug products, tamper-evident packaging requirements for, 172–174
Part 11 regulations, 84–85
  compliance, 76
  Subpart B, 85
  Subpart C, 85
Penicillin contamination, 181
Performance capability (P_p and P_{pk}), 124
Performance Qualification (PQ), 67
  of computer controls, 78, 78*t*
  table of contents, 67*t*
Personal computers (PCs), 81, 82*t*
Personnel factors, associated with CGMPs
  qualifications, 154–155
  responsibilities, for CGMPs, 155
  sanitation and health habits, 155–156
Plumbing, 26, 158
Preventive maintenance programs, 69–70
Process Analytical Technology (PAT), 67–68, 72
Process capability (C_p and C_{pk}), 124
  significance of, 127*t*

Process control, 165
  application programs, source code for, 29
  charge-in of components, 166–167
  deviations, 165–166
  equipment identification, 167
  in-process materials and drug products, sampling and testing of, 167–168
  microbiological contamination, control of, 168–169
  reprocessing, 169
  time limitations on production, 168
  written procedures, 165–166
  yield calculation, 167
Process development, 9, 87, 91*f*
  monitoring parameters, 92*t*
  process limits, setting, 99–101, 100*f*
  process parameters, 97–99, 98*f*
  risk assessment, 93–97, 93*f*, 94*t*
Process limits, setting, 99–101, 100*f*
Process metrics, 125
Process parameters, 97–99, 98*f*
Process Performance Qualification (PPQ), 10, 90–91, 103, 123
  executing, 109–112, 110*f*
    results, recording, 111–112
    sampling plans, 111
    validation report, 112
  preparing, 106–109, 108*f*, 109*t*
  process model, 107*t*
  protocol test ranges, setting, 104–106, 105*f*
  table of contents, 107*t*
Process Qualification (PQ), 9, 101
Process validation (PV), 5*f*, 6*f*
  beginning of, 47–48
  change control, role of, 35–37
  changes, types of, 37–40, 38*f*, 39*f*
  defined, 3–7
  documented evidence, 3–4
  example, 46–47
  flow of, 55, 55*f*
  life cycle approach, 33–35, 34*f*
  organization chart for, 45*f*, 46*f*
  protocol. *See* Process Performance Qualification (PPQ)
  requirements, for drug products, 29
  risks in, 4–5
  scientific evidence, 5
  stages of, 9–12, 11*f*
  wish list, 48, 49*t*
Process validation guideline—2011, 5
Process verification, continued, 104
Production, 165
  data, collection and evaluating, 119
    continued process verification, 125–126

control charts, 126–129, 127*f*, 127*t*, 128*f*
  legacy products, 123–125
  statistical process control (SPC), 126–129,
    127*f*, 127*t*, 128*f*
  record review, 18–19, 186
  time limitations on, 168
Product release, for distribution, 18–19
Programmed logic controllers (PLCs), 80–81,
    81*t*
Prospective validation, 7
Protocol generation error (PGE), 114–115
Proven acceptable range (PAR), 99–100, 104

Q
Qualification protocol execution, 68–70, 68*t*
  calibration, 69–70
  preventive maintenance programs, 69–70
  reports, 69
Quality by Design (QbD) program, 15, 30
Quality control unit, responsibilities of, 18,
    104, 154
Quality Programs, 53, 53*t*

R
Radio Frequency Interference (RFI), 78*t*
Random Access Memory (RAM), 76–77
Retrospective validation, 7
Returned drug products, 189–190
Revalidation, 7
Rinse method, 140
Risk(s)
  assessment, 93–97, 94*t*
    ICH Q9 approach, 93, 93*f*
  -based approach, 54–55
  management, 16, 30
  in process development, types of, 94*t*

S
Salvaged drug products, 190
Sanitation, 158–159
Sewage and refuse, 158
Short Change Control Form, 191
Site acceptance test (SAT), 55–57, 60–62
Software
  CGMP applicability to, 29
  functional testing of, 78*t*
  qualification, 73–74

Source code, 74–75
  for process control application
    programs, 29
Stable process, 122*f*
Standard Operating Procedures
    (SOPs), 35, 39, 111–112, 126
  preparation, 52
Statistical process control (SPC), 126–129,
    127*f*, 127*t*, 128*f*
Supervisory Control and Data Acquisition
    (SCADA), 83
  qualification, 83*t*

T
Time limitations on production, 168
Toilet facilities, 158
Total Organic Carbon (TOC), 139
Traceability Matrix (TM), 35
Training programs, 53–54
Trend analysis, 125

U
Unstable process, 122*f*
User Requirements (URS), 35

V
Validation master plan (VMP), 45, 48–52
  diagrams, 52*t*
  table of contents, 51*t*
  types of, 48
Ventilation, 25–26, 157–158

W
Warehousing procedures, 175
Washing facilities, 158
White box testing, 74
Wish list, for process
    validation, 48, 49*t*
Worst case situation, determining, 137, 137*t*
Worst case testing, 107
Written procedures, for production/process
    control, 17, 165–166

Y
Yield calculation, 167

Printed in the United States
By Bookmasters